NARRATIVE SOLUTIONS IN BRIEF THERAPY

The Guilford Family Therapy Series
Michael P. Nichols, *Series Editor*

Recent Volumes

NARRATIVE SOLUTIONS IN BRIEF THERAPY

Joseph B. Eron
Thomas W. Lund

THE GUILFORD PRESS
New York London

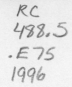

© 1996 The Guilford Press
A Division of Guilford Publications, Inc.
72 Spring Street, New York, NY 10012

Printed in the United States of America

This book is printed on acid-free paper.

Last digit is print number: 9 8 7 6 5 4 3 2 1

Library of Congress Cataloging-in-Publication Data

Eron, Joseph B.
    Narrative solutions in brief therapy / Joseph B. Eron and
Thomas W. Lund. — (The Guilford family therapy series)
    Includes bibliographical references and index.
    ISBN 1-57230-126-0
    1. Family psychotherapy.   2. Brief psychotherapy.
3. Strategic therapy.   4. Psychotherapist and patient.
I. Lund, Thomas W.   II. Title.   III. Series
RC488.5.E75   1996
616.89'156—dc20   96-2355
                                                                                CIP

Preface

This book was written to present the integrative approach to psychotherapy developed over the past 15 years at the Catskill Family Institute (CFI). During this time we have worked closely with colleagues trying to figure out how to help people overcome problems. Along the way we shared our ideas with others through dialogue, workshops, and journal articles. The format of a book afforded the scope to give a comprehensive account of our assumptions about how problems develop at different stages of the life cycle and how to resolve them.

The first three chapters describe the theoretical roots of the narrative solutions approach and give credit to the innovators whose ideas have shaped how a great number of psychotherapists help people. In Chapters 4 through 7, we present our assumptions about how problems evolve and the steps taken to help families reach narrative solutions. Chapters 8 through 13 address the practical applications of this approach to working with people across the life span. Chapters 14 and 15 highlight the special considerations taken in working with families in intense conflict, and how to talk with clients mandated for treatment or evaluation by social agencies.

This book represents not only the thinking of Joe Eron and Tom Lund, but also CFI clinicians Tim Adams, Steve Dagirmanjian, Jill Dorsi, Chris Farrell, Barry Garneau, Craig Lennon, Linda Rizzi, and Ken Russell, along with others who have trained and worked with us and have seen thousands of clients of all ages presenting with a range of problems, occurring at different stages of the life cycle. Their conversations with families in distress became our laboratory, and our conversations with them, grappling for solutions, and figuring out what worked and what didn't, became the basis of our approach.

Before Joe opened CFI in 1981, he was privileged to spend a day observing therapy and supervision at the Family Therapy Institute in

Washington, D.C. He sat behind the one-way mirror and watched as Jay Haley devised creative suggestion after suggestion to aid family therapists in training in their efforts to help families in trouble. Joe noticed that artificial time limits around numbers of sessions and work hours weren't reinforced. Therapists stayed with their families until there was movement toward change and supervisors stayed with the therapists until the job was done. At the end of a long day Haley was still eager to talk about ideas long into the evening. This passion for helping people overcome problems was an inspiration to Joe in starting CFI, and has carried on to the present.

In the 1980s, our close friend and colleague Michael Rohrbaugh provided a regular forum for us to present new ideas at the College of William and Mary in Williamsburg, Virginia. Michael's thoughtfulness about our work and his encouragement had a great deal to do with our interest in sharing ideas beyond the walls of CFI. At the annual Family Therapy Network Symposium, Richard Simon offered a venue for us to present new ideas about effective reframing. We'll never forget a hair-raising taxicab ride with James Coyne after our 1989 Network Symposium presentation in which we debated the merits of prescriptive and nonprescriptive practices in therapy. This conversation set the stage for expanding our thinking about the broader social context that shapes how people view and act around their problematic situations.

Upon Jim Coyne's recommendation, James Duvall invited us to teach at a unique externship program in Ontario, Canada. Jim Duvall had developed a training program that gives participants an opportunity to compare and contrast different brief therapy approaches by leaders in strategic, solution-focused, and narrative therapies. At a time when the emphasis in the field was in-with-the-new, out-with-the-old, Jim promoted integrating ideas in brief therapy. He contributed not only to our thinking about how to help people, but also to how to teach other therapists through workshops and presentations. His support for our integrative approach to brief therapy led to his introducing us to, among other people, Insoo Kim Berg and Michael White.

Insoo Kim Berg influenced our thinking as we reviewed CFI and solution-focused videotapes, highlighting similarities and differences between our approaches. As Insoo posed a frequent question, "How do you do that?," she challenged us to break down the elements of what we were doing that worked. We were struck by Insoo's total lack of interest in who did what better, and her passion for helping people change. Our conversations with Michael White inspired us to be clear in this book not only about what works but also about our own principles—what we believe in.

In the process of writing this book, we were fortunate to be invited to a gathering in Saratoga, California. Thanks to the efforts of Pat Emard of the Mental Research Institute and James Keim of the Family Therapy Institute in Washington, D.C., the "Unmuddying the Waters" meetings were held with about 30 people, some well-known pioneers in the field of brief therapy and newer colleagues like ourselves. Although seriously ill, John Weakland was an active participant, offering words of guidance for those who will be shaping the course of things to come in the field. A few weeks before his death, John Weakland wrote a letter to the *Family Therapy Networker* commenting on what transpired in Saratoga.

> The meeting explored common premises and values shared at a general level despite differences, and avenues of cooperation and collaboration to present to colleagues and students. While not always easy, one of the strengths of the field from its earliest days has been constructive reflection and discussion of its diversity. The emphasis on having things "my way" and needing something new each year has distracted us from serious and useful dialogue about what aids people in distress and facilitates change. (1995, p. 16)

John Weakland called for dialogue based on what's helpful to people, not on which school of therapy happens to be in favor this week and out of favor the next one. In a letter following the meeting in Saratoga, Pat Emard offered excerpts of advice from the original leaders in the family therapy movement. Weakland's advice was simply put. "Stay curious," he said.

It's in the spirit of integration and curiosity that we've written this book. We hope we've given credit where credit is due. We don't want to suggest that we have all the answers or that there is one correct way to do effective psychotherapy. Helping people change is a process of ongoing exploration.

Acknowledgments

We'd like to thank our close friends and business partners, Tim Adams, Steve Dagirmanjian, Ken Russell, and Craig Lennon, for their financial and emotional support in writing this book, as well as their thoughtful suggestions. Tim's creative work with people having substance abuse problems, Steve's innovative efforts with couples and adults, Ken's commitment to working with children and families, and Craig's compassion for clients experiencing trauma and abuse were an inspiration.

Our gratitude also extends to our dedicated support staff. Carole Sue Freer, Colleen Phillips, Heather Kubler, Karen Janitz, and Brenda Gogger set the tone for how people are treated at the Catskill Family Institute, speaking respectfully to clients seeking assistance and lending warmth to a hectic work environment. Thanks also to Jennifer Schmidt for her help in editing case transcripts.

Joe would also like to thank Susan Connors, the love of his life, for her unwavering support, and his children, Sarah and Bobby, for their tolerance and great title suggestions.

Tom would like to thank his wife, Mary Ann Sherman, and his daughter, Aimei, for their love and support throughout this project, and acknowledge William P. McDermott, Ph.D., who has had a profound effect in shaping Tom as a person and as a psychologist.

Our good fortune of having Michael P. Nichols as our editor for this book should not be overlooked. It was a privilege to have one of the most skilled writers in our field, and foremost authority on approaches to psychotherapy and family therapy, help us articulate our ideas and bring out our best.

Contents

NARRATIVE SOLUTIONS IN BRIEF THERAPY

Introduction

Our collaboration grew out of a shared curiosity for what helped people overcome problems. Tom was trained as a school and child psychologist and I (J. B. E.) could see that he had a special talent for talking with children, parents, and teachers in helpful ways. We met when Tom attended a talk I gave about the Mental Research Institute (MRI) brief therapy approach at a mental health center in our community.

In 1981 I opened the Catskill Family Institute (CFI) in Kingston, New York, and built the clinic around a brief systemic philosophy. Although open to other family therapy approaches, I was drawn to the simplicity and practicality of the MRI method. All therapists working at CFI heard more than their fair share about "problem cycles," "problem-maintaining solutions," and "symptom prescriptions" and more yet about the technique of "reframing," which had captured my fascination. The book *Change*, written in 1974 by MRI writers Paul Watzlawick, John Weakland, and Richard Fisch, achieved bible-like status in our group, and we all cited mantras from it. The phrase "Go slow" was heard a lot at staff meetings, and we perhaps too routinely warned our families and each other about the dangers of improvement.

Having an interest in learning more about the MRI method and systems thinking in general, Tom asked if I would supervise him. We used the one-way mirror, worked together on difficult cases, and soon found that the more we talked about our families, the better they did. After a while boundaries blurred and it became unclear as to who was supervising whom. That was all well and good. More troublesome was that certain systemic concepts that I held as near gospel were being seriously challenged by our results.

Tom, along with Tim Adams, joined me as codirectors at CFI in 1985. Later Steve Dagirmanjian, Ken Russell, and Craig Lennon also became partners. As the partnership expanded, so did the clinical services we provided. Between partners and full-time clinicians, CFI provides therapy for people experiencing a wide range of symptoms along life's path.

Over the course of 13 years of collaboration, Tom and I looked closely at what transpired between CFI's therapists and the families they tried to help. We observed that some of our conversations with clients were helpful. As they shed their problems, they came to see themselves, important others in their world, and their confining predicaments in new ways, ways that fit more comfortably with who they wanted to be. Other conversations weren't so helpful. Clients listened respectfully to what we had to say and tried new ways of doing things, but their views of self and other remained frozen and their situations were unchanged.

As we tried to sort out the difference between conversations that worked and those that didn't, we discovered some general principles for how to conduct helpful conversations with families in trouble. In the process we observed that problem resolution had less to do with the kinds of problems people presented or even the severity of their distress. Whether people got beyond their difficulties had more to do with the nature of the talks we had with them. There was something about helpful conversations that transcended aspects of persons or situations.

The ideas we present in this book about how to talk with people in distress also have important implications outside the treatment room. How parents talk to teachers, how teachers talk to parents, how bosses talk to employees, how doctors talk to patients, how child-welfare investigators talk to families under investigation, or how lawyers or mediators talk to divorcing couples can make or break an emerging problem and shape the course of things to come. While we'll touch on the impact of these conversations with families, this book will focus mainly on conversations that therapists have with people who come to them for professional help.

A CASE THAT CHANGED OUR THINKING

Early in our collaboration, we met a family that helped clarify our thinking about what worked in therapy. The family included 13-year-old Timmy, his stepfather, Vern, and his mother, Alice. Young Timmy had grown fond of testing Vern's authority as the "new father" in the family, prompting the family to seek help. Timmy was failing in school, mocking his teachers, setting school records for detention and suspension, fighting with school authorities, teasing his 4-year-old brother into tearful frenzies, and generally acting bratty.

What had been a warm relationship between Vern and his stepson soon became more like a series of scenes from the movie *The Great Santini*. Like Lt. Colonel Bull Meecham, Vern related to his teenage son as if he were a raw recruit at a Marine bootcamp. At the family's worst point, Timmy behaved badly, Vern resorted to drill-sergeant tactics to bring his behavior under control, and Alice looked on in exhausted exasperation. If Alice stepped in to comfort Timmy, seemingly interfering with Vern's discipline, Vern felt undermined and his tactics grew even harsher. If Alice supported Vern, Timmy looked at her with dismay, and she felt she had betrayed her son.

Here was a situation for an eager family therapist to sink his teeth into. The problem-maintaining cycle was easy to see. The more Vern tried to control Timmy's behavior, the more Timmy defied him. Alice's attempt to protect Timmy from Vern only nursed more bad behavior. When we discussed this case at our staff meeting, the voice of systemic reason echoed throughout the room. One staff member wondered whether young Timmy's symptoms were protecting Vern and Alice from facing their new marriage and their fear of intimacy based on past disappointments. Another proclaimed how Vern's attacks on Timmy served to protect the close bond between mother and son by driving her to rescue him. At that time in the development of our thinking, we'd shift back and forth between these different ways of looking at families in distress. Sometimes we'd look at problems in families with the idea of *homeostasis*, that symptoms served a purpose in keeping the system stable. At other times we'd simply look at *problem-maintaining solutions*, what people were doing about problems to keep them going. We didn't fully appreciate how these different perspectives about problem development implied different actions in the therapeutic conversation. We tend to talk differently with people when we think of them as cogs in a homeostatic system, than if we assume they are reasonable people whose well-intentioned efforts to solve their problems fall short.

AN UNHELPFUL CONVERSATION

I thought this classical family predicament could be easily mended by tried-and-true techniques. I didn't see any evidence that Timmy's symptoms served a particular function in diverting conflict between his parents, or in keeping their marriage together. My idea was to simply reframe Timmy's actions and intentions. By assigning a different meaning to Timmy's motives, I hoped to challenge Vern to act differently and inspire the couple to take a more unified approach to managing Timmy's behavior.

The new frame I offered was that Timmy was feeling a bit insecure about having too much power in the family. This was a familiar MRI refrain, but I tried to give it a unique twist to fit this particular family. I suggested that Timmy was afraid that history might repeat itself and that his parents wouldn't hold together as a unit. His rebelliousness, I said, was an attempt to test their unity. I tried to challenge the rigidity of Vern's drill-sergeant approach by suggesting that Timmy saw him as out of control, not calm and in command, and that this perception contributed to the boy's misbehavior. Alice nodded, seeming to agree with my assessment. Still stonefaced, now slumping into his chair, Vern made no comment.

Then, the discussion turned to disciplinary tactics that the parents might agree on to help Timmy feel more secure. As I had hoped, Alice and Vern came up with more reasonable consequences for misbehavior, but their commitment to change seemed thin. There was no ring of conviction in the conversation to lend confidence that a pattern had been broken.

There was some improvement, however. Vern eased up on the extreme punishments and agreed with Alice on more reasonable consequences for misbehavior. Timmy's behavior and schoolwork improved, and more often than not, he did what was asked of him at home and at school.

Although Vern went along with the changes made, he never really altered his mistrustful view of Timmy and always seemed about ready to explode. He frequently slipped back into old behavior patterns. After a setback occurred, Alice would arrive at the next therapy session rolling her eyes in disgust, as Vern sheepishly admitted to another blowup. After several more sessions, the parents again reported some improvement and said they had decided to take a break from therapy. This decision seemed to have more to do with weariness than satisfaction with our results.

The family came back 1 year later in even more distress. Timmy was staying at a temporary shelter for runaway children, and Vern and Alice were considering a more permanent placement outside of their home. Alice requested that Timmy see a child psychologist; Vern cast his vote for military school. Tom and I talked this over, and Tom suggested that he meet with Timmy alone and interview Vern and Alice. Then we'd present our ideas to the parents. Timmy returned home during this three-session "evaluation."

A HELPFUL CONVERSATION

After Tom's meetings with family members, we both sat down with Vern and Alice, having carefully prepared what we would say. I watched and listened as Tom explained how young Timmy saw his world. Much of what was being said fell outside of our prepared spiel. Worse yet, it sounded a lot like individual therapy talk. I controlled my discomfort by reminding myself that Tom was just building up to the strategic reframe that we devised in advance.

Tom went on about the early days in Vern and Timmy's relationship, noting how Timmy looked up to his stepdad. He said that Timmy was impressed with all the things that Vern could do, his success at work, his athletic prowess, and his ease at fixing things around the house. As I listened, I realized that Tom wasn't making any of this up. He used actual quotes from his conversations with Timmy; his sincerity was obvious. He seemed to know and like this young man and had respect for his view of things. As the conversation progressed, I also couldn't help but notice changes in the mood in the room. As Tom spoke about how Timmy actually saw his stepfather, Alice smiled warmly. She seemed to agree with this positive portrayal of Vern, looking as if all she wanted was for Vern and Timmy to recapture what they once had. Contrary to our clever systemic speculations at the staff meeting, this did not look like a woman invested in an overprotective relationship with her son or someone motivated to stay distant from her husband. I glanced over at Vern. He, too, looked different. The stern glare and stonefaced demeanor that prevailed in our conversation 6 months earlier had all but disappeared. Vern looked animated. Leaning forward in his chair, he seemed pleased with what was being said and eager to hear more.

Tom continued. He talked about the trouble Timmy was having living up to his stepdad's image. Like most boys approaching their teenage years, he said, Timmy was struggling with questions about his awakening identity. Who am I and who will I become? What will the rest of my life be like? These were the large questions on Timmy's mind. Will I turn out to be more like my real father, a failure and confirmed troublemaker? Or, will I be more like my stepfather, a solid citizen whom people look up to? Tom described how Timmy was trying to reconcile this new "improved" father who was not his flesh and blood with the old father who shared his genes but drank heavily, treated his mother badly, couldn't hold a job, and ultimately walked out on the family.

As Tom talked, the mood in the room shifted. Alice looked sad; Vern was subdued; both of them seemed caught up in this story about their son. They seemed to join in compassion for Timmy's predicament and were actually mulling over a new explanation for his outrageous behavior.

I now awaited the punch line, the zinger, the "strategic" part of the conversation that Tom and I had prepared ahead of time and that we hoped would jolt the parents out of their frozen positions. Tom gazed over at Vern and said that sadly, and with the best of intentions, Vern had been helping Timmy out with his theory about men. Timmy was, in fact, beginning to see Vern as the spitting image of his genetic father, even though *we* all knew that he was nothing like him. He had somehow lured Vern into behaving like his father by acting as if he didn't care much for Timmy and by declaring that he wanted him out of the family. Timmy's theory about how fathers behave was being confirmed.

As we had hoped, this reframing of current events did light a fire under Vern. Vern gazed at Tom intently. The dialogue went as follows:

VERN: Hold everything. What can I do about this theory?

LUND: Well, we didn't really plan on what you should do about that. We talked about seeing what your reaction would be and what we could come up with together.

VERN: I don't know. Maybe we're going to need to outsmart him, since he's been outsmarting me. You think I'm going to have to be nice to the boy?

Alice looked stunned, but she offered little resistance. I felt as if I could hear her muttering under her breath something to the effect of "Nice to the boy? Nice to the boy? That'll be the day."

LUND: Why would you be nice to him?

VERN: Well, he's been doing this and that to get me to punish him, and I guess I'll have to be nice to him to outsmart him.

The session ended, with Vern launched on a mission to show Timmy his true colors as a father and to straighten out Timmy's twisted theory about men being uncaring and rejecting. And he prevailed despite Timmy's best efforts to dissuade him.

Alice and Vern began to support each others's efforts at discipline, which became far less severe and nonblaming. Vern seized every opportunity to rekindle the warmth and caring in his relationship with Timmy. Gradually, Timmy's behavior improved, both at home and in school, and his grades shot up. Therapy ended 5 months (12 sessions) after Tom's first session with Timmy. Three years later, Tom ran into Alice at the local mall. Alice said that Timmy's grades were still excellent, and he was working part-time and helping his stepdad renovate the house the family had purchased. A new story of the family had replaced the old one, and talk of problems had all but vanished.

The difference between what happened in the room with these two parents on this occasion and what happened 1 year before was like night and day. Why on this occasion did Vern become actively engaged in the dialogue and in the sincere search for solutions? Previously he just listened passively, going through the motions. What was it about the earlier conversation that failed to move him? And what about the difference in Alice's reaction? In my contact with the family the year before, Alice seemed to join with me as I described Timmy seeing Vern as an out-of-control father. This time she seemed to join with Tom as he described Vern as a loving father whom Timmy looked up to. She welcomed Vern's effort to get back to what he and Timmy once had. Then there was the question about Timmy's participation in the therapy. My knowledge about Timmy came from conversations with his parents about him. I didn't get to know Timmy as a person or understand his views about himself, his family, or his situation. When I suggested alternative motives for his outrageous behavior, did the parents question the authenticity of my comments?

Because Tom really got to know their son, did Alice and Vern have more confidence that he knew what he was talking about? Were the individual sessions with Timmy just a prelude to the real therapeutic action, that is, the strategic reframing that was offered the parents? Or, did we really learn something about Timmy's inner world that helped us understand more about the problem and about how to talk to the parents to make it better?

Our thinking about what worked in therapy developed as we tackled questions like these. None of these factors alone accounted for why one conversation was helpful and the other was not. In the helpful conversation, however, past, present, and future dimensions of family life were tapped in a way that touched people's emotions, brought out their compassion for each other, and inspired them to find creative solutions to their entrenched predicament.

Families like Timmy's taught us a great deal about what went into therapeutic conversations that produced change. In the process of refining our ideas about what worked, our thinking about human problems—their evolution, their continuation, and their resolution—went through major revision. We can now explain what was helpful in talking with this family far more precisely than we could have 10 years ago. But to do this we had to tamper with the traditional ways that strategic therapy was being practiced and part somewhat from the orthodoxy of the times.

—JOSEPH B. ERON

—1—

The 1970s and 1980s: An Emphasis on Action

The 1970s brought an infusion of bold new ideas about families and how to help them change. Many of these concepts had their roots in Gregory Bateson's famed research project on communication, which took place in Palo Alto, California, in the 1950s. The Bateson project assembled many of the brilliant thinkers that came to shape the field of family therapy. At that time there were no circumscribed schools, no opposing theoretical camps, no restrictive allegiances to stifle creative thinking. Imagine renowned communicators such as Milton Erickson, Virginia Satir, John Rosen, R. D. Laing, and Don Jackson being studied by keen observers such as Jay Haley, all trying to decipher the knots of disordered conversation and clues to untie them. Out of this collection of curious minds came groundbreaking ideas that shaped much of our thinking about families and psychotherapy. At the time, these ideas shook the foundations of traditional thinking about human problems. To these pioneers, "schizophrenese" was an intelligible language that made sense in the context of family communication rather than being the mad babbling of thought-disordered individuals. Traditional conceptions of psychopathology were stood on their heads. Behavior once seen as abnormal or aberrant was now regarded as adaptive to its particular context.

Ironically, it was Gregory Bateson, an anthropologist, a man wary of tampering with people's lives, who wound up founding the culture of family therapy. He did this by introducing systemic thinking, or what he called the "epistemology of pattern," into the field (Bateson, 1972, 1979). Doing therapy systemically meant looking for pattern, difference, process, and relationship. The intrinsic characteristics of individuals—personality traits, biological predispositions, unconscious

9

conflicts, and social skills—became secondary to the ongoing communicational patterns in which their lives were embedded.

Bateson taught therapists to think in circles rather than lines. The clinical syndrome of depression, for example, couldn't be understood in isolation from the repetitive actions of others involved in communication around the despondent person. The whole pattern of interaction around expressions of despondency had to be considered for depression to be fully explained. Problem and pattern were inseparable. This concept of circular causality helped family therapists make startling discoveries. We found that serious symptoms could be alleviated by changing the patterns of interactional behavior that sustained them. The idea that these symptoms could be the exclusive property of one person came to be questioned. It was more like the symptoms were on loan, contained within a relational context that created and nurtured them.

An outgrowth of the Bateson project, the Mental Research Institute (MRI), was opened in 1961 under the direction of Don Jackson. One of the first productions of this group was an intriguing book entitled *Pragmatics of Human Communication* by Paul Watzlawick, Janet Beavin, and Don Jackson (1967). Criticized by Bateson for inaccuracies and omissions, and for drifting into the suspect arena of interpersonal influence, this work nonetheless became the inspiration for the development of future models of family therapy. *Pragmatics* captured some of the eclectic magic of the Bateson project, exploring realms beyond therapy. The authors delved into philosophy, narrative, and literature, and wrote a compelling communicational analysis of Edward Albee's great play *Who's Afraid of Virginia Woolf?*

If you read *Pragmatics* for the first time, you'll experience the excitement of the early days of family therapy, when bold ideas about the nature of human problems were being shaped. If you reread this book from the vantage point of the 1990s, you'll see connections to the narrative therapy movement, which has recently captured the attention of the field.

SCHOOLS OF FAMILY THERAPY EMERGE

In the year 1974, the brief problem-focused therapy approach, developed at MRI, was first presented in an important book entitled *Change: Principles of Problem Formation and Problem Resolution* by Paul Watzlawick, John Weakland, and Richard Fisch. Later, their work was summarized in a seminal article (Weakland, Fisch, Watzlawick, & Bodin, 1974). In that same year, Salvador Minuchin introduced the field to a bold new approach which he called structural family therapy (Min-uchin, 1974). In 1976, Jay Haley, who worked at MRI in the 1960s and joined Minuchin at the Philadelphia Child Guidance Clinic in 1967, published a work entitled *Problem Solving Therapy*, which combined MRI and structural influences (Haley, 1976). By the time Haley and Cloé Madanes opened the Family Therapy Institute of Washington, D.C., in 1976, his thinking tilted more toward Minuchin's structural/ organizational concepts and away from MRI's problem focus. This shift became obvious with the publication of the book *Leaving Home* at the close of the decade (Haley, 1980).

Haley (1980) often made the point that the chief value of systems theory was that it taught therapists to recognize repeating sequences and make predictions. In structural approaches, circular sequences usually involved at least three people and were the basis for inferring anomalies in organizational structure. Haley and Madanes became concerned with hierarchies, with who was up and who was down in the family structure, and with how confusion or incongruity in this arrangement shaped problems. Thus, with severely disturbed young people trying to negotiate the difficult transition of leaving home, a therapist might look for sequences in which "the parent told the youth what to do, but he did not do it, or the parents did not tell the youth what to do but complained about what he did, or the youth told the parents what to do and the parents did it" (Madanes, 1980, p. 190). Other problem sequences were viewed as indicators of a confused hi-erarchy in which covert coalitions crossed generational lines. Thera-pists trained by Haley and Madanes were taught to notice times when a parent or grandparent nurtured a child after another parent attempt-ed discipline, and to develop strategies to change these sequences.

Structural family therapists promoted the notion of homeostasis. Symptoms were seen as serving a function in maintaining the stability of the family unit. In Haley and Madanes's model, a young person poised to separate from his or her parents might develop "mad" or "bad" behavior to protect the existing family order and prevent the leaving home transition from taking place. Subtly, an assumption of negative intention seeped into structural explanations of the family impasse. The young person, somehow sensing that his or her parents might have trouble with the transition at hand, acted disruptively. The parents, having trouble shifting to a new family structure without the young person, rallied around his or her symptoms to keep the family hierarchy intact.

Whereas Haley's writing emphasized the vertical dimensions of structure, Minuchin highlighted the horizontal aspects. Minuchin's concepts of enmeshment and disengagement emphasized how close or distant family members were from each other, and how their relative proximity affected the course of problems. The idea that symptoms served a function came through, but in a different form. For example, a young person's symptoms might be seen as preserving closeness between a mother and son, as maintaining a father's distance, or as blocking intimacy or conflict in a disengaged marriage. The connection made between the symptom and the organization that surrounded it caused structural family therapists to think they had to intervene actively and forcefully to rearrange family structure.

In Minuchin's approach, directive intervention might mean choreographing who talked to whom or who sat next to whom in the family session. Intervention might also involve actively challenging patterns of transaction as they occurred in the room, or giving the family a task that brought a "disengaged" father into direct contact with his children and helped an "overinvolved" mother move out of enmeshed conversations. In the approach of Haley and Madanes, the therapist might insist that parents come together with a plan to manage the "lazy" behavior of an adolescent son whom they saw as "crazy." Or, the therapist might arrange for parents to take charge of discharge planning with a troubled young person who had been hospitalized.

Minuchin and Haley had different styles. Minuchin used his warmth and commanding presence to grapple with people in the room. He enjoined and engaged, then challenged people to alter their rigid ways of talking and relating to each other. His style was up close and personal. In contrast, Haley's strategic approach kept him more removed from the family. Haley was more a student of therapy than an enthusiastic practitioner. He'd sit attentively in the calmer quarters of the room behind the one-way mirror and there devise a strategy to help an exasperated young therapist disentangle from an unproductive interaction going on in the therapy room. The therapist conducting the session would pick up the phone and listen to Haley's succinctly delivered, respectful advice about what to do next. The advice would be in the form of a creative directive.

To Minuchin, the therapist was a mover and shaker, pushing the system into a new order while it tried to stay the same. To Haley, the therapist was the consummate, somewhat aloof strategist, arranging ways for the system to shift into a new order while it tried to remain stable. Both men felt that therapists had to be active and directive intervenors in order to dislodge a stuck symptom from a stuck system. Although their styles were different, they shared a common philosophy about the structural basis of symptoms, and about the therapist's responsibility for engineering change.

While problem-focused and organization-focused approaches were being developed in this country, an ultrasystemic, ultrastrategic approach was being crafted in Europe. A group was formed in Milan, Italy, by child psychiatrist Mara Selvini Palazzoli that included Selvini Palazzoli, Luigi Boscolo, Gianfranco Cecchin, and Giuliana Prata. Paul Watzlawick of MRI consulted with the group in its early days, showing the intimate link between these emerging schools.

The Milan group expanded upon the methods pioneered at MRI, in particular, the use of the therapeutic double bind, or what they referred to as the "counterparadox." In their first book, *Paradox and Counterparadox*, published in 1978, the Milan group introduced their most compelling technique, "positive connotation." Typically, the entire problem situation affecting the family would be positively reframed by the therapist or therapeutic team and the family warned against premature change. In this book, the authors describe such an intervention with a 6-year-old boy, his 3-year-old brother, and his parents (Selvini Palazzoli, Boscolo, Cecchin, & Prata, 1978).

At the close of the session, to enhance the dramatic impact of the message and to minimize disqualifying feedback from the family, a letter from the team was read aloud to everyone. In the letter, young Bruno, the identified patient, was praised for acting crazy to protect his father. By preoccupying his mother's time with fights and tantrums, the boy generously allowed his father more time for work and relaxation. Bruno was then encouraged to continue doing what he was already doing, lest this comfortable arrangement be disrupted.

With the technique of positive connotation, the Milan group put yet another twist on the idea that symptoms served a function to protect the system from the uncertainties of change. Although the behavior of the identified patient was typically recast as generous and protective of the system's integrity, there was often the negative implication that others benefited from that protection. Imagine being the parents of a schizophrenic youth, who are told that your child's madness was needed to keep you intact. This hardly suggested to the parents that their own intentions were positive.

Lynn Hoffman, commenting on the work of the Milan team, suggested that they were influenced by the Bateson project's inquiries into game and coalition theory, which grew out of the Cold War (Boscolo, Cecchin, Hoffman, & Penn, 1987). Cold War language appeared in the Milan team's description of the therapist's struggle with a recalcitrant family system. The homeostatic forces that were working to keep the family frozen in time had to be countered by the carefully coordinated tactics of the therapeutic team, some of whom had to sit behind a one-way mirror to avoid being drawn into the family's entangling web. To change, the family had to be outmaneuvered, outwitted, and outflanked.

THE INFLUENCE OF MILTON ERICKSON

While these schools of strategic, structural, and systemic family therapy were developing, an important solitary figure was working behind the scenes, significantly shaping the zeitgeist. Although he never identified himself as a family therapist, the late Milton Erickson profoundly moved the field. Haley studied Erickson's techniques of hypnotic communication after being introduced to him by Bateson in the 1950s. Haley's writings about his work brought Erickson's imaginative ideas into the growing field of family therapy (Haley, 1973, 1985a, 1985b, 1985c).

In one of his many tributes to Erickson's inspirational genius, Haley introduced Erickson as the first strategic therapist, then corrected himself and referred to Erickson as the first therapist, period. Haley regarded Erickson as the only major clinician of our time whose life's work was devoted to changing people. Prior to Erickson, Haley said, clinicians spent much of their time pontificating about the pathogenic workings of the human mind and developing intricate coding systems for describing abnormal behavior. Erickson's main concern was with helping people, and he came up with some ingenious ways to incorporate people's own ideas in the service of solutions. Erickson had little concern with allegiances to individual or family therapy. Sometimes, he'd meet with individuals, sometimes with couples, sometimes with the whole family—whatever got the job done.

The main link between Erickson's innovative work with hypnosis and his influence on strategic family therapy was the introduction of what he called the "utilization principle"—using the client's language as a way to minimize resistance in therapy. Using this technique, Erickson was able to induce trance in suggestible or nonsuggestible hypnotic subjects. With this innovation, he helped to alter the idea that resistance was contained within the person, and promoted the idea that it melted through the medium of a well-managed therapeutic conversation. Erickson made it clear that it was the therapist's job to figure out how to talk with people so that resistance disappeared.

We'll expand upon Erickson's original ideas about the art of therapeutic conversation as we describe our own approach. These include the strategic use of language, the importance of appreciating people's preferences and of joining them "where they're at," and the technique of seeding new ideas with people that are a natural extension of their own worldviews.

Erickson will probably always be remembered, however, as the quintessential strategic therapist. Perhaps one of his most important contributions had to do with emphasizing the therapist's responsibility for change. In many ways he transformed what case conferences were all about. Old saws about the patient being "too resistant," "questionably motivated," or "too psychiatrically unstable" to change were met with questions about courses of action. What do you plan to do to reduce resistance, to increase the patient's motivation, and to help the person to act more stable? These became common retorts at strategic therapy case conferences. With Erickson, therapists became experts in the arena of creating change rather than experts on why people stayed the same. Therapists became men and women of action.

Perhaps Erickson's most controversial legacy to family therapy had to do with the use of uncommonsensical techniques (see Haley, 1973). In seeing and helping thousands of patients, Erickson developed a variety of unique strategies for producing change, which included paradoxical prescriptions, symptomatic ordeals, unusual task assignments, and uncommon responses to common client complaints.

AN UNCOMMONSENSICAL APPROACH

For example, Haley (1973) described a conversation between Erickson and a 16-year-old girl who sucked her thumb compulsively, to the exasperation of her parents, teachers, and schoolmates. She was told by the school psychologist that her thumbsucking was an aggressive act. In the session, the girl removed her thumb from her mouth and declared to Erickson that she didn't like "nut doctors." Erickson decided to utilize the girl's aggressive inclinations by giving her an unusual task. He said:

> The only thing I'm interested in is why, when you want to be aggressive about thumbsucking, you don't really get aggressive instead of piddling around like a baby that doesn't know how to suck a thumb aggressively. What I'd like to do is tell you how to suck your thumb aggressively enough to irk the hell out of your old man and old lady. (p. 195)

Erickson, in a resolute tone of voice, then instructed the girl:

> Every night after dinner, just like a clock . . . go to [your] father's favorite sitting place in the living room and really nurse [your] thumb good and loud and irk the hell out of him for the longest twenty minutes he has ever experienced. (p. 196)

As a condition of taking the case, Erickson had already arranged with the parents to back off completely from saying or doing anything about the thumbsucking, and to let Erickson supply the cure. Each night for the next few evenings the girl was faithful to her performance. Then it began to irk her to have to be so irksome to her parents. She began to shorten the time, then began late and quit early, then skipped, and finally forgot about it altogether. In less than 4 weeks the girl stopped sucking her thumb, both at home and elsewhere. Erickson altered a lifelong habit in one session.

Unfortunately, when reading about these dramatic improvements, many therapists wanted to run right out and try the same thing with a similar problem. To their disillusionment, the techniques didn't work. So, they'd go right back to doing what they were doing before, now convinced that they weren't clever enough to become brief therapists.

These uncommon techniques became the calling card of strategic family therapy, more so than the basic principles upon which they were predicated. For adherents of the strategic approach, it was said that if a problem could be solved "without the family knowing how or why," that was sufficient (Madanes, 1980). Given Erickson's pragmatic bent and disinclination to explain what he did in precise theoretical terms, his techniques were open to all sorts of possible interpretations, leaving plenty of room for misapplication. There seemed no question that Erickson knew exactly what he was doing. But for many practitioners trying to follow in his large footsteps, it seemed that if a problem could be solved without the therapist knowing how or why, that too became sufficient. Attention was drawn to the magic of techniques rather than the methods of therapeutic conversation. In this spirit of technique worship, the more manipulative side of strategic therapy got noticed. Lost were the gems about language and how to talk respectfully with people in change-producing ways.

A COMMONSENSICAL APPROACH

Let's contrast Erickson's application of the utilization principle with the thumbsucking case with his approach to a young woman from New England who was injured in a car accident (see Haley, 1973). She was embroiled in an endless round of lawsuits, which placed her in the role of a handicapped person. She stopped exercising, working, socializing, and having fun. Erickson hypnotized and regressed the young woman back to the time before her accident, when she was in private school. He inquired about what she learned there, noting her achievements. He then shifted her attention to the future, inviting her to talk about what she wanted to do after all the lawsuits and quarrels were behind her. She began to talk about marriage and having a family, imagining herself following in the footsteps of an older sister who'd just had a baby. It was Easter time and Erickson asked the young woman if she ever heard of a New Englander enjoying swimming in the winter, then suggested she try the pool when she got back to the motel. Feeling invigorated after this *different conversation* with Erickson, she took him up on the suggestion and enjoyed the experience. Apparently, this event set the stage for change because the young woman gradually broke away from acting handicapped.

In the thumbsucking case, Haley remarked that Erickson commanded the girl's attention through an aggressive tone that matched her own. He also caught her attention by using language such as "old man" and "old lady," presumably to enlist her resistance in the paradoxical service of the therapeutic directive. The idea was to redirect the girl's defiance in a way that challenged the family's current patterns of interaction. Presumably, once the symptoms stopped serving a useful propose, they'd go away. It wasn't clear, however, that Erickson had aligned with the girl's preferences and intentions. Was her preference to be defiant? Did she view thumbsucking as an achievement or life aspiration?

In the car-accident case, Erickson applied the utilization principle differently. He helped the young woman look back to a time when she was acting in line with who she hoped to be, when she was active in school and still learning. He invited her to think toward a future free of a handicapped mind-set. This emphasis on preferences and positive intentions had more appeal than the focus on paradoxical prescriptions in the thumbsucking case. As you'll see, highlighting preferred views and integrating past, present, and future experience are basic to our approach.

Erickson's use of uncommonsensical techniques became a prominent feature of the MRI brief therapy approach. But it wasn't to the use of these surprising, paradoxical techniques and unusual prescriptions that we resonated. The simplicity, practicality, and inherent optimism contained in MRI's assumptions about the nature of human problems and their resolution became the basis of the development of the CFI approach in the mid-1980s.

—2—

From MRI to CFI:
Linking Meaning
and Action

In the mid-1980s, we took a close look at clinical applications of the MRI approach, studying what MRI-trained therapists said and did with families. We zeroed in on their key assumptions about how problems evolve, persist, and resolve.

The first assumption concerned the origin of problems. Problems developed from the mishandling of ordinary life difficulties, which usually occurred at key transition points in the life cycle (e.g., marriage, divorce, birth of a child, separation, major illness, children leaving home, death). Problems were not necessarily caused by dysfunctional persons or systems; nor did they serve a purpose in keeping families intact, regulating boundaries, or maintaining power arrangements.

These ideas about the formation of human problems were not fully developed by strategic therapists, whose primary concern became changing the immediate interaction that surrounded and maintained symptoms. However, the notion that problems were likely to crop up during times of normal transition in the life cycle was a major theme in the writings of other leading family therapists of the 1970s and 1980s (e.g., Haley, 1973; Carter & McGoldrick, 1980). The CFI approach elaborates on this concept of the innocence of problem evolution. As you'll see, tracking how problems evolve from the points of view of family members caught in stuck predicaments is one of the keys to solutions.

A second important MRI concept that influenced our approach involved the persistence of problems. The well-intentioned attempts of family members to solve problems actually maintained problems. The therapist's job was to figure out what people were doing about their difficulties that kept them going, then to devise a strategy to get them to act differently.

The third MRI assumption involved the resolution of problems. Problems were resolved simply by interrupting problem-maintaining behaviors and getting people back on course, on to and over the next hurdle in life. Typically, this was done by influencing people to take a new course of action, something other than their more-of-the-same problem-solving attempt.

These three principles implied that people could get into problems with the best of intentions, and could get out of problems without a major overhaul to either their personality structures or family structures. Therapists could enter conversations with people in distress without feeling as if they had to move against an immoveable force (homeostasis) that was holding everyone back from change. Change wasn't a forbidding prospect that people resisted. Therapy could be elegantly simple.

MRI CASE EXAMPLES

Let's look at two MRI case examples that illustrate how these assumptions were applied in therapy. You'll note that we use a concept called the "problem cycle" to explain how MRI therapists approach problems and solutions (see Rohrbaugh & Eron, 1982; Eron & Lund, 1993). We portray these problem cycles using circular diagrams to pinpoint the therapist's strategy for change.

> In a frequently cited MRI case (Watzlawick & Coyne, 1980), a therapist sat down with the wife and grown children of a depressed stroke victim who attended only the first session. The man, from everyone's description, saw himself as being the head of the household until the stroke left him helpless. Family members, trying hard to be helpful, cheered him up, gave him encouragement, and did lots of things for him, only to find that he became even more withdrawn and despondent. Taking into account the family members' shared view of the patient as being proud and stubborn, the therapist *reframed* his depression as the last refuge of his pride and self respect, then *prescribed* a series of tasks designed to get family members to act more helpless in his presence. As the family took on this new approach, they began to report a positive change in the man's overall mood and activity level.

Based on this case description, we'd portray the problem-maintaining cycle in a circular diagram. Figure 2.1 illustrates a more-of-the-same behavior pattern. The more the stroke victim acts depressed, the more family members try to help and encourage him. With repetitions of this cycle, problematic behaviors persist and intensify (see Figure 2.2).

Problem Cycle

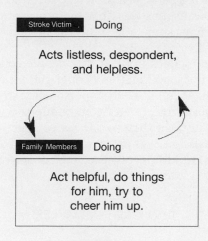

FIGURE 2.1.

Problem Cycle

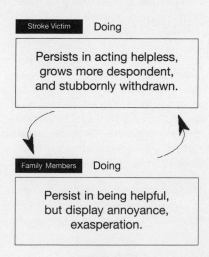

FIGURE 2.2.

Solution Cycle

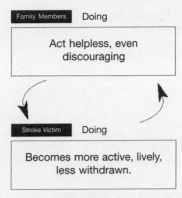

Family Members Doing

> Act helpless, even
> discouraging

Stroke Victim Doing

> Becomes more active, lively,
> less withdrawn.

FIGURE 2.3.

Equipped with this formulation, the therapist planned an intervention to reverse the problem cycle by influencing people to behave differently. We'd portray the solution in another circular diagram. Figure 2.3 illustrates a less-of-the-same behavior pattern. The less family members try to help (or more helpless they act), the less depressed the stroke victim acts. With repetitions of this positive feedback loop, the presenting problem resolves (see Figure 2.4).

Solution Cycle

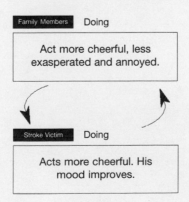

Family Members Doing

> Act more cheerful, less
> exasperated and annoyed.

Stroke Victim Doing

> Acts more cheerful. His
> mood improves.

FIGURE 2.4.

Interestingly, MRI cases often involved treating only one person, as in the next example.

> In a case in which a woman was experiencing obsessive rumina-tions, the patient was seen as trying hard to rid herself of disturb-ing thoughts. But the more she tried to bring the thoughts under control, the more the thoughts seemed to control her, and a more-of-the-same cycle ensued. The therapist took into account the pa-tient's preference to be in control of her life in assigning an unusu-al task. She was told to try to bring on the negative thoughts at scheduled intervals during the day as a way to enhance her con-trol over them. She was also advised to have the thoughts when she was usually not bothered by them and to keep them in her mind even as they tried to leave (Fisch, Weakland, & Segal, 1982).

Here, we'd portray the problem cycle using a similar circular dia-gram. Figure 2.5 also shows a more-of-the-same behavior pattern. The more the client tries to eliminate intrusive thoughts, the more she ex-periences the bad thoughts. Thus, the problem cycle persists (see Fig-ure 2.6).

Once again, the purpose of therapeutic intervention was to alter this problem-maintaining cycle. The therapist assumed that if the client tried to bring on the bad thoughts, her experience would be dif-ferent. Her thoughts would become less alien, less intrusive, and less preoccupying, and her sense of self-control would be reclaimed. We'd

Problem Cycle

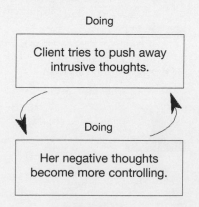

FIGURE 2.5.

Problem Cycle

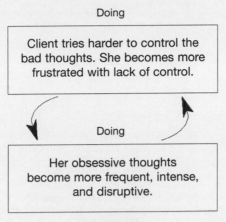

Doing

| Client tries harder to control the bad thoughts. She becomes more frustrated with lack of control. |

Doing

| Her obsessive thoughts become more frequent, intense, and disruptive. |

FIGURE 2.6.

map this solution cycle with another circular diagram (see Figure 2.7). As the client reversed her problem-solving approach, a positive feedback loop was set in motion. Paradoxically, the less the client tried to control the negative thoughts, the less the thoughts exerted control over her. With repetitions of this solution cycle, her situation improved (see Figure 2.8).

Solution Cycle

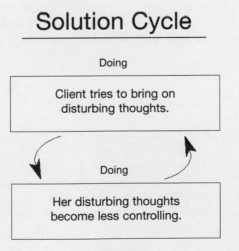

Doing

| Client tries to bring on disturbing thoughts. |

Doing

| Her disturbing thoughts become less controlling. |

FIGURE 2.7.

Solution Cycle

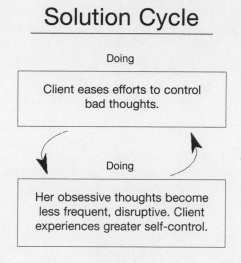

Doing

Client eases efforts to control bad thoughts.

Doing

Her obsessive thoughts become less frequent, disruptive. Client experiences greater self-control.

FIGURE 2.8.

Although there was nothing in the basic assumptions of the MRI approach to suggest this, we observed that in the vast majority of MRI case illustrations problem cycles were thought of in behavioral terms. The emphasis was on action—figuring out what people were doing in the present that maintained problems and influencing people to behave differently to resolve problems. Family members' views were taken into account only to promote compliance with a behavioral task or directive. The role that meaning played in the evolution and maintenance of problems and their resolution went largely unnoticed.

VIEWING *AND* DOING

We realized early on in our application of MRI concepts that we weren't comfortable with the prescriptive aspects of the treatment approach. We felt ill at ease persuading people to do things that we wanted them to do but that they often didn't want to do. We were far more interested in the neglected "viewing" aspects of people's experiences, and how these experiences were linked to problem-maintaining behavior.

The constructivist underpinnings of the MRI approach were articulated by Paul Watzlawick, who authored several books on the subject of meaning, including *The Invented Reality* (1984), *The Language of Change* (1978), and *How Real Is Real?* (1976). In all these accounts, consideration was given to the idea that meaning was socially constructed, that truth was relative, and that reality was invented, not discovered. Watzlawick (1984) distinguished between first-order realities that had to do with the properties of objects, and second-order realities which had to do with meaning, significance, and values—the stuff of human affairs. "Relationships," he said, "are not aspects of first-order reality, whose true nature can be determined scientifically. Instead they are pure constructs of the partners in the relationship, and as such they resist all objective verification" (p. 238). Watzlawick reminded us that the "map is not the territory; the name is not what it names; an interpretation of reality is only an interpretation and not reality itself. Only a schizophrenic eats the menu instead of the foods listed on the menu" (p. 215).[1]

In an interesting elaboration of Watzlawick's constructivist ideas to the process of problem maintenance, Jeffrey Bogdan (1986) emphasized the connection between meaning and action. "It cannot strictly be the case," he said, "that behaviors, problematic or otherwise, are maintained by other behaviors. I have no access to your behavior per se, only to my representation, or interpretation of it. Therefore, it must be my interpretation of your behavior, not your behavior per se, that maintains my own actions" (p. 35). In terms of actual clinical practice, the only foray that MRI therapists made into the realm of meaning came through the application of an intriguing technique called "reframing." By experimenting with this technique, we developed ways to merge the realms of meaning and action, that for all practical purposes had been kept separate from each other.

---

[1]Paul Watzlawick is widely recognized for introducing constructivism to the field of family therapy (Watzlawick, 1984). The technique of reframing, also introduced by Watzlawick and his colleagues at MRI and popularized by strategic family therapists, is often linked to constructivist principles. Social psychologist Kenneth Gergen is generally regarded as the leader of social constructionist thinking, often embraced by narrative therapists (Gergen, 1985). The technique of restorying is often tied to this philosophy. Although distinctions have been drawn between these schools of thought, we do not emphasize these differences in this book (see Gergen, 1985; Efran & Clarfield, 1992). Instead, we show how reframing and restorying can be used together. Our approach is based on tracking how individual and social constructions, embedded in dialogue between people, are linked to problems; and how alternative constructions, embedded in conversation, are linked to solutions. Also consistent with social constructionist thinking, we view the therapist as responsible for generating and managing helpful conversations inside and outside the treatment room.

THE ART OF REFRAMING

The technique of reframing was first introduced to the field of family therapy in the book *Change* (Watzlawick et al., 1974), which devoted a forward-looking chapter to what was called the "gentle art of reframing." At that time, reframing was defined as a way "to change the conceptual and/or emotional setting in which a situation is experienced and to place it in another frame which fit the 'facts' of the same concrete situation equally well or even better, and thereby changes its entire meaning" (p. 95).

In practice, this gentle art of reframing soon became the clever art of therapeutic persuasion and salesmanship. In the book *The Tactics of Change*, which came out in 1982, reframing and redefining were "commonly, although not exclusively, used means for getting clients to adopt a course of action they would otherwise refuse to take" (Fisch et al., 1982, p. 119). As in the previous case examples, in which a woman plagued by intrusive thoughts was persuaded to bring them on at scheduled intervals, or the overly helpful family members of a depressed man were invited to act helpless in his presence, reframing became a way to get people to go along with unusual therapeutic prescriptions or tasks.

There were, however, exceptions to this practice. Reframing was not always the handmaiden of a behavioral directive; sometimes, a reframe stood alone and was used to change how people viewed their own behavior and the actions of others with whom they were caught in problems. For example, there was the familiar case of a pursuing wife and distancing husband in which the therapist told the wife that her nagging behavior was protective of her husband. By sacrificing her own image, he said, she was helping him look good in the presence of others. With this redefinition, the therapist softened the meaning of nagging, placing it in a context of sensitivity and protection, which suggested that the wife's intentions were positive and well meaning (Watzlawick et al., 1974).

We were left wondering, however, whether this reframing fit the facts of the marriage; whether a general theme of nurturance, overresponsibility, and protection pervaded a range of interactions between the couple; or whether patterns of pursuit and distance had special meaning to the couple even before they entered the marriage. We were left to assume that this reframing fit somehow within a broader context of meaning that rang true for the couple, but we were given only the faintest outlines of the larger story. Somehow, by inverting the meaning of the wife's nagging behavior within the narrow confines of the couple's current interaction, they found new ways of relating.

How or why remained a mystery. Did the wife suddenly shift gears because the last thing she wanted to do was make her husband look good? Did the husband actually alter his view of the wife's behavior, now seeing her as more sensitive and less critical of him? With this change in perspective, did he begin to pursue her more, thus breaking the cycle?

FROM MAGIC TO METHOD

Whether reframing was used to change a view or sell a do, the problem with strategic applications of reframing was that they were often arbitrary. It wasn't always obvious what views were being altered and how these views were linked to the pattern of behaviors that the therapist was trying to change. One of MRI's own researchers, James Coyne (1985), recognized these shortcomings and became interested in expanding the understanding of reframing. He noted that the therapeutic use of reframing, which was basic to strategic therapy, lacked an adequate conceptual scheme for explaining what worked. In order to provide viable reframes, he suggested that therapists acknowledge key aspects of patients' existing frames and link reframes to them. For reframes to endure, they must anticipate and somehow be validated in patients' ongoing interactions with their everyday environments. Coyne also reminded us that frames were created, perpetuated, and altered in a social or intersubjective context. We are dealing with interactional processes, he said, that could not be reduced to the thought of a single participant. Coyne was advocating what we later called a "cognitive-interactional" approach to problems, in which reframing could be used effectively (see Eron & Lund, 1989).

C. Wayne Jones (1986) commented on the wide use of reframing among family therapists, yet noted that there was little discussion about what factors actually motivated family members to accept new frames. Although seasoned clinicians might have developed an intuitive understanding of these factors, others were left to apply reframing tactics in an ad hoc manner, often guided by erroneous assumptions. It wasn't uncommon, he said, for trainees

> who attempt to learn reframing strictly from reading case studies in the family therapy literature or from attending brief technique-oriented workshops to conclude that the strategy is limited to a set of brilliant, catchy statements delivered by the therapist which have instant "magical" effects on families. They seem to assume that reframing is some "thing" administered "to" a client-system. (p. 58)

Jones suggested that training of family therapists could be improved if experienced clinicians spent more time showing what was done to make clever reframes appear sensible to families and explained how new frames were woven into the ongoing therapeutic conversations.

A NOT-SO-ARTFUL REFRAME

Our own experience taught us that blind imitation of the technique of reframing sometimes produced unhappy results.

We remember the case of a frail 9-year-old boy who refused to speak. His sister and parents assumed the role of ventriloquists and did all his talking for him. We told his reserved parents, who valued good manners, that the boy's symptoms were a sign of discourtesy and disrespect. By making the problem one of manners, we hoped to motivate the parents to help the boy begin talking for himself, thus interrupting their problem-solving attempt. We thought this was pretty clever, and we anticipated one of those magical turnarounds so famous in the annals of strategic therapy. Instead, the parents stiffened in their seats and looked more demoralized than mobilized. From their point of view, we were being disrespectful by not appreciating the boy's delicate nature and by maligning their good intentions as parents. Like the expression on their faces, their view of the situation remained frozen, and we retreated sheepishly to our offices to work on *our* manners.

Mistakes like this one made us think twice about waving a therapeutic wand and pulling a reframe out of the hat. Simply twisting the meaning of behavior by arbitrarily relabeling craziness as laziness, madness as badness or sadness, or symptoms as assets, was not enough. Although we might have wished it were so, frogs could not so easily be turned into princes.

As James Coyne remarked, it was important to understand the existing views of people who come to us for help. We became interested in tracking how these views became connected to the problem over time. Perhaps the reframe that developed from this careful assessment would make sense to people. The new frame might fit plausibly within a system of meaning that shaped their own actions, yet jostle the fit in a purposeful way, so that new actions emerged. As C. Wayne Jones suggested, reframing need not be some "thing" that we imposed on people to convince them to follow our directions. Effective reframes should emerge as we talk with people about their predicaments and attempt to explain things differently.

Although our purpose in therapy remained to disrupt problem-maintaining, more-of-the-same behavior, we moved to a broader consideration of people's views of self and other as they converged on their present predicament. We became intrigued by certain questions that were unanswered in our scrutiny of MRI cases. For example, in the case of the stroke victim, the idea that he was a "proud and stubborn" man came to be known through conversation with family members. How, we wondered? Did this preference have something to do with how the problem got started in the first place? Did he view himself historically in the family as someone who was more the helper than the helped? When family members started to offer solicitation and encouragement following the stroke, did he begin to regard himself differently? Did his increasing despondency have something to do with an increasing conviction that his family now saw him as helpless and ineffectual? When family members began acting helpless, did he become reacquainted with his old helpful self and reconsider the actions and intentions of others from a more self-confirming perspective?

We asked these kinds of questions as we moved further into the realm of meaning, and the important part it played in the evolution, maintenance, and resolution of problems. We will address these questions in the next chapter.

—3—

The 1990s: An Emphasis on Meaning

As we were exploring the link between meaning and action around problems and solutions, a major shift in thinking and practice was occurring in the field of family therapy. Postmodern therapies, based in narrative and social constructionist principles, were evolving. The watchword was meaning. Narrative therapists were talking about meaning with the same zealous fervor that strategic therapists had talked about action a decade before. The field had entered a new era.

SOLUTION-FOCUSED THERAPY

New schools of family therapy were proliferating. In Milwaukee, Steve de Shazer and Insoo Kim Berg developed a bold new approach called solution-focused therapy which, like our own, had its roots in the MRI brief therapy approach (Berg & de Shazer, 1993; de Shazer, 1985, 1991). However, their therapy is based on a shift in focus away from talk about problems and toward talk about solutions. In a departure from MRI, solution-focused therapists say little about how problems arise and what interactions between people keep problems afloat. The emphasis is on helping people locate strengths and resources to effect change in their lives.

Solution-focused therapists inquire more about what people are doing when the problem doesn't occur than when it does occur. This search for *exceptions* to problems is the basis for much of the therapeutic conversation. A compelling technique called the "miracle question" situates clients in a future vision of life without the problem, encouraging people to describe in some detail what they will be doing differently once they are problem free.

The solution-focused approach altered how therapists converse with families. Therapists are taught to notice competencies, not deficiencies; solutions, not problems. In keeping with the MRI approach, the emphasis is on behavior, on what people do differently that results in solutions. Solution-focused therapists tend not to inquire deeply into the meaning that people derive from these successful occasions in life. The question of how exceptions reflect on people's views of themselves and others close to them is largely unaddressed.

Still, solution-focused therapists consider language and meaning to be basic to therapeutic change. "As the client and therapist talk more and more about the solution they want to construct together, they come to believe in the truth or reality of what they are talking about. This is the way language works, naturally" (Berg & de Shazer, 1993, p. 9).

The solution-focused approach carries the MRI approach's spirit of minimalism and elegant simplicity into the 1990s. It's not necessary to change intrapsychic structures or family structures, or even to change redundant behavioral patterns. Therapists need simply to help clients talk differently about their lives, and to notice their own successes.

THE HOUSTON–GALVESTON APPROACH

In Houston, Texas, Harlene Anderson and the late Harry Goolishian (Goolishian & Anderson, 1987) developed an approach based on social constructionism. To these innovators, "Problems are no more than a socially created reality that is sustained by behavior and coordinated in language" (p. 532). As they put it, the problem determines the system more so than the system determines the problem. Those persons who are most touched by the problem constitute the system, and so form the unit focused on in therapy. The problem is defined, not as an objective entity but as a shared construction that shapes what we, the observers, come to call the system. Therapy is a process in which therapist and family co-create new narratives that "dissolve" problems, and in which the therapist is first and foremost a "manager" of conversations. Anderson and Goolishian (1992) portrayed the therapist as coming from a "not-knowing" position, a far cry from the take-charge, expert position of the strategic therapist.

Many of the catchwords of the narrative therapy movement come from the writings of the Houston–Galveston group, such as "co-created meanings," "collaborative dialogue," a "nonimpositional therapeutic stance," "nonhierarchical conversation," the "not-knowing position" and problems "dissolving" rather than being solved. In large part, this new language is about humanizing the process of therapy, bringing the therapist down off the lectern and making him or her a part of the conversation.

THE REFLECTING TEAM

Some of the new narrative therapies move even further away from focusing on the immediate problem, away from what people are thinking and doing to maintain it, and away from talking to people about what to do to get beyond it. A good example is an innovation, the reflecting team, introduced by Norwegian therapist, Tom Andersen. Andersen's work is influenced by recent developments in the Milan approach. By the late 1980s, Milan therapists shifted from talking about systems as essentially stable and homeostatic to describing them as ever changing, evolving, and only appearing to be static (see Tomm, 1984a, 1984b). This notion about families as evolving "meaning systems" grew more popular.

The reflecting team is a postmodern contrast to detached observers sitting behind the one-way mirror designing strategic interventions. The team sits right down in the room with the family and comments directly, face-to-face, on what they observed. Different permutations and combinations of reflection are possible. The team might reflect on what they observed, the family might reflect on the team's reflections, and the team might then reflect on the reflections of the family. As Andersen (1991) emphasized in the subtitle of his book, there are "dialogues and dialogues about the dialogues."

MICHAEL WHITE AND DAVID EPSTON

In contrast to narrative therapists in North America and Europe, Michael White, at the Dulwich Centre in Adelaide, Australia, and David Epston of New Zealand, remained problem focused. Yet these therapists spoke about problems and therapy in a profoundly different way than their predecessors or contemporaries. From the idea of thinking of people as "having problems," they moved to the idea of problems "having people." Problems were oppressive, alien invaders that took over people's lives and prevented them from being who they wanted to be.

White and Epston (1990) observed that as problems come to dominate people's lives, the stories they tell about themselves become negative and "problem saturated." *Externalizing conversations* are designed to separate persons from problems and help them marshal their own resources against problems. Therapists invite clients to map the effects of the problem on their lives, which helps them notice the problem's tyrannical influence and organize against it.

For example, White (1989) offered an example of mapping the influence of "Sneaky Poo" (a name given the problem) on the lives of an encopretic child, Nick, and his exasperated parents, Sue and Ron. In doing so, the family discovered the following:

1. Although Sneaky Poo always tried to trick Nick into being his playmate, Nick could recall a number of occasions during which he had not allowed Sneaky Poo to "outsmart" him. There were occasions during which Nick could have co-operated by "smearing," "streaking" or "plastering," but he declined to do so. He had not allowed himself to be tricked into this.
2. There was a recent occasion during which Sneaky Poo could have driven Sue into a heightened sense of misery, but she resisted and turned on the stereo instead. Also, on this occasion, she refused to question her competence as a parent and as a person.
3. Ron could not recall an occasion during which he had not allowed the embarrassment caused by Sneaky Poo to isolate him from others. However, after Sneaky Poo's requirements of him were identified, he did seem interested in the idea of defying these requirements. . . .
4. After some discussion, it was established that there was an aspect to Sue's relationship with Nick that she thought she could still enjoy, that Ron was still making some attempts to persevere in his relationship with Nick, and that Nick had an idea that Sneaky Poo had not destroyed all of the love in his relationship with his parents. (pp. 10–11)

Note in this example how the problem of encopresis is given the name "Sneaky Poo" and how the family is enjoined to outsmart him. The therapist shifts the influence from the problem to Nick, Sue, and Ron, helping them to notice their own resources to overcome the problem.

In White's approach, one of the therapist's main jobs is to help people get in touch with *unique outcomes*, aspects of lived experience that fall outside of the dominant "problem-saturated" accounts of their lives. Unique outcomes include times when the problem is not present or when the person acts in line with preferred ways of being.

The search for unique outcomes is similar to the solution-focused therapist's emphasis on exceptions to the problem. However, White and his colleagues encourage people to talk about the meaning behind their stories and their experience of events, while also helping people notice their own successes. Once located, these unique outcomes are plotted by the therapist and family into an alternative story or narrative. For example, in the case of Nick, Ron, and Sue, and their struggle with Sneaky Poo, White also invited family members to "reauthor" their lives and relationships. He went about this by asking people key questions. "How had they managed to be effective against the problem in this way? How did this reflect on them as people and on their relationships? Did this success give them any ideas about further steps that they might take to reclaim their lives from their problems?" (p. 11).

Michael White and David Epston provide a map for the therapist to navigate an effective conversation. There's purpose to the therapist's comments and questions, and a direction to the search for alternative stories. White and Epston view therapists as accountable for what they do. Although the client is seen as the expert and primary author, and the therapist is the secondary author in the restorying process, it's the therapist who assumes primary responsibility for change. Therapists restory with the specific aim of deconstructing the problem, changing its meaning, and loosening its hold over people's lives.

As the major architects of the narrative therapy movement, White and Epston have humanized family therapy. They've brought the person back into the system—by affirming that an individual's preferences, intentions, stories, and experiences are relevant to the process of change. Like strategic family therapists of the 1970s and 1980s, however, these postmodern therapists have a plan for changing problems.

RESTORYING *AND* REFRAMING

As we reflected on the contributions of narrative and solution-focused approaches of the 1990s, we reexamined what we were doing with families we treated. It wasn't simply that key views of self and other maintained repeating cycles of behavior in the present. These views were also embedded in significant stories from the past. History played a part in the construction of problems and informed how we talked with families to generate solutions. Our forays into the realm of meaning had taken us from "reframing" to "restorying," techniques we've come to see as compatible and as simply applicable to different contexts of meaning.

In practice, reframing was applied to the immediate interactional context that surrounds the problem. The term "frame" was used by

Bateson (1972) and later Goffman (1974) to define the narrow range of meaning that encompassed the current situation. The analogy of a picture frame was used to show how psychological frames include certain messages and exclude others.

Let's return to the case of Timmy, Vern, and Alice described in the Introduction to illustrate how the concepts of frame and story are compatible, and how the techniques of reframing and restorying work well together. You may recall that 13-year-old Timmy began failing in school, arguing with his parents, fighting with school authorities, and generally acting bratty. Timmy's stepfather, Vern, viewed his behavior within the frame of "disrespect."

Vern saw Timmy as disrespecting him and mocking the authority of adults in general. Once Vern fixed on this frame, he ignored exceptions to this pattern. Should Timmy act considerately toward friends, teachers, or his mother, while still acting disrespectfully toward him, Vern would cling to his existing frame rather than attempt to reconcile the contradiction or entertain an alternative frame. Perhaps he'd forget past occasions when Timmy was "good," or even if he did recall these times, he might *explain* these exceptions in a way that maintained the "bad" frame. People stuck with fixed problems are usually stuck in fixed frames through which they can only see how to do more of the same.

The narrow frame within which Vern thought of Timmy affected how Vern acted toward Timmy. Vern resorted to drill-sergeant tactics, harshly trying to control Timmy's misbehavior. The more punitive Vern acted, the more disrespectful Timmy acted and the more evidence Vern acquired to support his negative frame.

When first introduced by the MRI group, reframing was a technique to alter how people viewed their current situation to change their behavior. You'll recall that in an early conversation with Timmy's parents, Vern and Alice, Joe attempted to reframe Timmy's behavior. He suggested that Timmy's rebelliousness was an attempt to test parental unity. Joe referred to a past event, Timmy's abandonment by his biological father, but didn't elaborate on its meaning to family members. He simply said that Timmy was fearful that history might repeat itself; that was why he was testing his parents' resolve to stick together as a unit. You may recall that this reframe fell flat. Although the parents tried to work together as a unit to set reasonable consequences for Timmy's behavior, their teamwork quickly disintegrated. They returned a year later to our offices in even more distress.

The second time around, Tom engaged in a different conversation with the parents, one that inspired rapid improvement. In a more helpful conversation, Tom incorporated information that family members had imparted about their *past* experiences, which shaped the way family members framed their current situation. Thus, the therapist *restoried* experiences of past events in a way that led to reframing present circumstances, using these two techniques together.

Whereas reframing applies to the current situation, restorying applies to a broader context of meaning that embraces past, present, and future dimensions. In introducing this technique, White and Epston (1990) describe a story or self-narrative as follows:

> In striving to make sense of life, persons face the task of arranging their experiences of events in sequences across time in such a way as to arrive at a coherent account of themselves and the world around them. Specific experiences of events of the past and present, and those that are predicted to occur in the future, must be connected in a lineal sequence to develop this account. This account can be referred to as a story or self-narrative. (p. 10)

Our work with Timmy, Vern, and Alice was more successful when we elaborated upon the meaning of past events in the context of present action. Tom spoke with both parents about a key view Timmy had about fathers. He learned about this view by talking with Timmy about past experiences with his biological father and more recent experiences with his stepfather. Tom emphasized how Timmy once held different views of the two men. He reminded the parents of the early days in Timmy and Vern's relationship, when there was fondness and warmth, and he emphasized Timmy's respect for Vern. When Tom then suggested that Vern's current behavior was supporting Timmy's worrisome theory about fathers, Vern listened intently. He quickly became motivated to disprove Timmy's troublesome theory and change how he was acting toward him.

In the helpful conversation, Vern began to reframe Timmy's behavior. He began to see positive intentions in Timmy's (negative) actions and notice his own contribution to Timmy's rebelliousness.

In later sessions with this family, a story of Vern's abandonment by his two daughters from a previous marriage was also drawn out. Thus, two stories of past abandonment were unveiled, and the meaning attached to these stories became relevant to the solution.

The therapist learned that Vern's view of past rejection by his daughters influenced his present interpretation of Timmy's disrespectful behavior, which in turn shaped his actions around that behavior. Another story about Vern's father and his remembered role as a strong disciplinarian and community leader also cast new light on the current interaction. Vern saw himself as failing to be the father he hoped to be, saw Timmy as disrespecting his authority, and saw his own father as being disappointed in him. This constellation of negative views helped construct the current frame within which Vern saw Timmy. Vern acted toward Timmy in a way that was in line with this father-as-failure frame.

This joining of restorying and reframing seemed far more effective than using one or the other technique alone. Reminding Vern of past exceptions, unique outcomes, or alternative stories without addressing the present circumstance or problem was a hit-or-miss proposition. Similarly, suggesting to Vern that Timmy was really insecure, not disrespectful, in an arbitrary manner that *did not* present a coherent account of their relationship over time, might also fall flat. Stories affect frames and frames affect stories.

RECOVERING THE GENTLE ART OF REFRAMING

Whereas we maintained an interest in the relationship between restorying and reframing (thinking that the reconstruction of meaning around current interaction was relevant to narrative therapy), other postmodern commentators were using harsh words to portray the technique of reframing. For example, Efran, Lukens, and Lukens (1988) described strategic therapists as playing "fast and loose" with language in applying reframes. In contrast to strategic therapists, these authors said they were constructivists, "interested in simplifying and demystifying life's problems, not in adding additional layers of counterintuitive, half-believed, poorly substantiated mumbo jumbo." They added that "there is a subtle but critical difference between taking liberties with established definitions and proposing fresh problem-solving frameworks" (p. 34).

Perhaps this critique was justified by the sometimes arbitrary ways reframing was used by strategic therapists in the past. In fact, we'd characterize Joe's initial intervention with Timmy, Vern, and Alice as an example of fast-and-loose reframing. However, we were concerned that reframing itself was being connoted as a *necessarily* manipulative and impositional technique.

Reframing, once heralded as a "gentle art" (Watzlawick et al., 1974), lost its gentility in the strategic practice of therapeutic prescription and persuasion. Yet, there was nothing manipulative about being purposeful in therapy, in altering meaning to change action, or in influencing people to overcome problems. These aspects of strategic practice were and are compatible with narrative concepts.

As family therapy entered the 1990s, it wasn't that the technique of reframing needed to be discarded. Nor did we need to abandon the emphasis on therapist responsibility intrinsic to strategic practice. What needed revision was the undue emphasis on salesmanship. Selling people on following a therapist's directive wasn't the only way to influence them to break loose from entrenched patterns. Guiding people to rethink their assumptions about problems and reconsider the actions and intentions of others important to them was a perfectly respectful and effective way to help people change. Thus, reframing remained a gentle art in the way we applied the technique, and one compatible with nonimpositional, narrative approaches to problems and change.

Effective therapeutic conversations enter the realms of story *and* frame; address meaning *and* action; and, by so doing, help to resolve problems. It's in mapping how the broad realm of narrative touches on the narrow confines of the problem cycle that creative solutions are best found. Although the problem may be a construction that dissolves through a well-managed conversation, the problem is nevertheless very real to the people affected by it. The problem, as our clients see it, is the basis of their pain and distress, and the reason they enter into conversation with us.

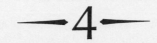

Toward a Theory of
Problem Construction

I n order to plan helpful conversations, it's important to understand
how problems are constructed. Steve de Shazer (1985), a proponent
of solution talk as opposed to problem talk, has acknowledged the
importance of clarifying one's own assumptions about complaint development. He stated,

> Therapists need to make some assumptions about the construction of
> complaints and the nature of solutions to do their job. . . .These assump-
> tions can be seen to operate like rules for mapping complaints and prob-
> lems. If a therapist uses a certain set of assumptions, say "Y," then a cer-
> tain type of map will develop. (p. 22)

In our approach, mapping how people become fixed on problematic views of self and other leads to an understanding of how the socially constructed reality they call the problem can be deconstructed.
Therapists needn't wander around in the narrative dark, not knowing
what stories to look for or what views to change. Paul Watzlawick
(1984) offered a useful social constructionist metaphor that depicts
how we see the haphazard, although not entirely accidental, route to
problem development.

> A captain who on a stormy night has to sail through an uncharted chan-
> nel, devoid of beacons and other navigational aids, will either wreck his
> ship on the cliffs or regain the safe open sea beyond the strait. If he loses
> ship and life, his failure proves that the course he steered was not the
> right one. One may say that he discovered what the passage was not. If,
> on the other hand, he clears the strait, this success merely proves that he
> literally did not at any point come into collision with the (otherwise, un-
> known) shape and nature of the waterway; it tells him nothing about

how safe or how close to disaster he was at any given moment. He passed the strait like a blind man. His course *fit* the unknown topography, but this does not mean that it matched it. (p. 14)

There is no precise route through life that steers us away from problems. We continue to bump against unforeseen obstacles along the way. It's the meaning we ascribe to these bumps, and to the actions of people affected by them, that determines our ultimate course. These ascriptions of meaning give shape and contour to our journey and lend to it some measure of predictability. Since there is no predetermined route to problems—or solutions—we must begin with people's own constructions and understand how they took shape to create the configuration of ideas and actions that constitute the problem. If we listen carefully to people we're trying to help and track their experience of events significant to them, we will arrive at an understanding of their own peculiar path into the straits of problem construction. Once we have this map, we, the navigators of the conversation, can help them steer back into the open seas.

An extremely articulate 14-year-old girl named Jean, whose independent spirit was being spent in seemingly endless battles with her father, helped shed light on this process of problem construction. We'll use her story to elucidate our assumptions.

PROBLEM CONSTRUCTION: A CASE OF UGLY ARGUING

When Jean's mother called to make an appointment, she defined the problem in terms of the "constant, ugly arguing" that went on between Jean and her father. Recently, their verbal battles had turned into pushing and shoving matches. Through tears, Mrs. Ryan spoke about her own feeble attempts to referee the two combatants and how this was tearing her apart. Lately she lapsed into siding with whomever seemed "least unreasonable," more often than not, her daughter. After all, she said, with just a hint of sarcasm, her husband was the adult and should have more self-control than his 14-year-old daughter. After several tries, Mrs. Ryan convinced her unyielding husband and defiant daughter to come to counseling to help her with *her* upset. Repeated attempts to convince the combatants that it was *their* problem hadn't worked.

In the first therapy session, family members related an example of a typical scene from their lives. Mr. Ryan came home from work and noticed Jean sitting on the couch eating popcorn and watching TV. She ignored him. Father commented, "I told you not to eat in the living room . . . besides, don't you have homework to do?" Jean sighed theatrically and continued to watch TV, deliberately not looking at her father. Finally she muttered, "Lighten up, Dad. Are you stressed out from work or what?" Mr. Ryan called Jean lazy and hopeless; she responded with an obscenity; Mr. Ryan started yelling; Mrs. Ryan entered the room and asked her husband to please calm down, saying, "You just walked in the door. Do we have to start in already?"

A typical evening in the life of the Ryan family had begun, culminating in everyone going off into their separate corners with an icy silence in the air. The only calm member of the family was Jean's brother, John, who managed to stay out of the fray. When things heated up, he'd talk to his friends on the phone or close his bedroom door and quietly do his homework.

This vignette typified a more-of-the-same cycle of behavior that perpetuated the problem. The more disrespectful Jean acted, the more Mr. Ryan yelled at her, and the more Mrs. Ryan criticized her husband for overreacting. The ensuing conflict promoted emotional withdrawal among family members, punctuated by outbursts of ugly arguing. By tracking this repeated sequence of behavior, the goal of therapy became clear.

If Mr. Ryan were to calm down and join with his wife to set realistic expectations for Jean's behavior, Jean would probably act less defiant and the ugly arguing would stop. This behavioral goal is similar to what a structural family therapist would look for in realigning the hierarchy or reinforcing system boundaries. The goal is also similar to what an MRI brief therapist would aim for in disrupting the father's problem-maintaining solution of coercion and exhortation.

After family members gave us a clear picture of the behavioral interaction, Jean asked the therapist an interesting question. "Dr. Lund," she said, "my brother did the same thing last week and nothing happened. I'd like to know why." She went on to describe how her brother was told to mow the lawn as soon as he came home from school. Instead, he invited some friends over to watch a tape of a basketball game, and they all ate sandwiches in the living room. Jean described how she waited around to watch the fireworks, expecting to see her brother get the brunt of her father's anger for once. To her dismay, Mr. Ryan didn't say or do anything about the matter. The following interaction ensued over the question of the father's nonreaction.

MR. RYAN: (*looking thoughtful*) I seem to remember that I did say something to John like, "You know you guys shouldn't be eating in the living room."

JEAN: Yeah. And that is all you said. You didn't *do* anything about it.

LUND: (*to Mr. Ryan*) Do you remember what John said to you?

MR. RYAN: Yeah. He said he was sorry and promised they would clean up when they were through.

JEAN: (*rolling her eyes*) But he was supposed to be mowing the lawn, and you never said anything about that!

MR. RYAN: I seem to remember that John apologized for forgetting to mow the lawn. Maybe that's why I didn't say anything. [John verified this story.]

JEAN AND MRS. RYAN: (*in unison*) But you let him eat in the living room, and he never did mow the lawn that day.

John remained quiet, while his father looked puzzled.

What emerged in this conversation was that everyone in the family agreed about a key difference. John did many of the same things that Jean did, but with very different results.

Objectively speaking, eating popcorn in the living room isn't much different from eating sandwiches in the living room, yet Mr. Ryan's *reaction* to the two situations was dramatically different. Obviously his contradictory response had something to do with how he *viewed* the two situations and the people involved in them. This relates to our first assumption about problem evolution and problem maintenance.

Assumption 1. How people feel and how they act in a situation depends on how they construe the situation.

This first assumption is about the self exclusively. It follows the thinking of personality theorist George Kelly. Salvatore Maddi (1968), in a comparative analysis of different theories of personality, wrote that "for Kelly, events have an actual existence separate from man, but do not achieve importance for understanding personality until they are construed by him" (p. 114). Ultimately, we must take into account how each individual caught in the web of problematic interaction *construes* the actions of others. In this case, Mr. Ryan's reaction to the event of eating popcorn in the living room set in motion the emotionally charged responses that followed.

To fully comprehend Mr. Ryan's construction of the event, however, we must consider how he viewed others around him. The event itself seems innocuous. The meaning father assigned to the event must be based on how he had come to see his daughter's actions and intentions, which was quite different from how he had come to see his son's actions and intentions. This leads us to our second assumption.

Assumption 2. A person's construction of an event or a situation, and consequently how he feels and how he acts, depends largely on his view of the other. This includes his construction of the other person's motivations and intentions and his view of the other's view of him.

R. D. Laing (1969) wrote extensively about how individual constructions about self and other affect family interaction. He observed that "the person whom we describe . . . is not the only agent in his 'world.' How he perceives and acts toward the others, how they perceive and act towards him, how he perceives them as perceiving him, . . . are all aspects of the situation" (p. 66). Laing and his colleagues previously described how a person's self-identity was a composite of his view of himself and his view of how others see him (Laing, Phillipson, & Lee, 1966).

Mr. Ryan's ideas about Jean's intentions contrasted with his ideas about John's intentions. He felt that Jean did things to "intentionally provoke him," that she had "no interest in cooperating," and that she clearly "disrespected" him. On the other hand, he saw John as "basically a good kid" who "cared" for him, "respected" him and valued his advice. Thus, his construction of how Jean saw him was very different from his construction of how John saw him. In his mind, his daughter regarded him as an unworthy father, undeserving of her respect, and his son saw him as a decent father whom he still valued. Obviously, John's apology for eating in the living room and Jean's sassy response reinforced these preexisting constructions.

Jean and her brother, John, filled the therapist in on their own ideas of Dad's behavior and shed more light on why he responded differently to the two eating incidents. With a hint of sadness in her voice, Jean said that her father treated her brother with far more "respect" than he treated her. As the therapist expressed interest in Jean's point of view, she burst into tears. "He thinks I'm stupid, or retarded, and he doesn't respect me at all as a person," she said. John chimed in with his perspective on the father–daughter conflict. He felt that neither one had respect for the other. "You're just like Dad," he said. "You can't let anything go. You know he can be picky. I just let it ride, and that's what you should do."

Now that we had these three perspectives on the two "eating" events and the people involved in them, we could explain why one situation triggered a problematic interaction and the other did not. Mr. Ryan's differing reactions were an outgrowth of differing viewpoints about Jean and John's actions and intentions, and how he felt they viewed him. Similarly, Jean's defiant behavior became more explainable once we understood her perspective about her father's actions and intentions and how she thought her father viewed her. John, too, helped us understand why Father's reaction to his eating sandwiches in the living room was so mild. Although he saw his father as "picky," he did not attribute any negative intention to his actions. He simply felt, "That's just him." Since he saw his father seeing him as a "good kid" who was competent and worthy of respect, he was better able to accept his father's ways.

The basis for the emotional intensity of people's reactions to events relates to the next assumption.

Assumption 3. People have strong preferences with regard to how they would like to behave, how they would like to see themselves, and how they would like to be seen by others. We refer to this constellation of ideas about self as a person's "preferred view."

This concept of preferred view appears in different shapes and forms in the writings of prominent self psychologists and family therapists. For example, the concept of preferred view was implied in the client-centered therapy developed by Carl Rogers, whose ideas bear a marked resemblance to postmodern, nonimpositional concepts about therapy and change. Rogers (1961) proposed that people experience distress when there is a gap between their ideal self and self as perceived. Successful therapy closes this gap. "During and after therapy," Rogers said, "the perceived self would be more positively valued, i.e., would become more congruent with the ideal or valued self" (pp. 234–235). William James (1890/1984) made a similar distinction between the "immediate and actual and the remote and potential selves" (p. 315).

More recently, Hazel Markus and Paula Nurius (1986) introduced the notion of "possible selves" to "represent individuals' ideas of what they might become, what they would like to become, and what they are afraid of becoming" (p. 954). Similar to our concept of preferred view, possible selves serve both a motivational and evaluative function. People are motivated to achieve their possible or desirable possible selves and to avoid their negative or undesirable possible selves, and evaluate their own behavior in relation to these standards. In our terms, we compare events in our lives against constructions of preference, and we're motivated to reconcile gaps between how we'd like things to be and how we think events turn out. Like our concept of preferred view, the concept of possible selves implies that there is no "real" singular representation of self. We're not describing schemas lodged inside our psyches, but rather a constellation of evolving possibilities by which we measure our life experience and construct who we are.

Strategic family therapists also recognized the therapeutic importance of understanding how people want or *prefer* to be seen by others. For example, in their seminal article presenting the MRI approach, Weakland, Fisch, Watzlawick, and Bodin noted that they determined early in treatment "what approach would appeal most to the particular patient—to observe where 'he lives' and meet this need, whether it is to believe in the magical, to defeat the expert, to be a caretaker of someone, to face a challenge, or whatever" (1974, p. 156). Narrative therapists Michael White and David Epston (1990), touching on the concept of preferred view, emphasized how "preferred outcomes" or "preferred stories" are drawn out in the course of therapeutic conversations to open up alternative possibilities for change. They noted that often these preferred stories and preferred outcomes were hidden, buried under "problem-saturated" accounts of the self. This clinical observation squared with the research findings of Markus and Nurius (1986), who pointed out that a person's possible selves are less obvious to other people than their active, "real" self-representations. Thus, people might act in ways that are out of sync with their own preferences, but their wishes might not be apparent to others they are close to. As you'll see in our case example, both Jean and her father ultimately reveal that they would like to have a close relationship. They're both unhappy, even saddened, by their current interaction. These preferences wouldn't be obvious, however, if one looked only at their current actions or listened to their problem-saturated accounts of their present situation.

Let's be clear that we do not see "preferred view" as a "thing" that people "have" and can't get rid of. Rather, we're talking about a host of possible views or preferences that suit people, that fit with who they wish to be. For example, "I'm clever," "I'm a good mother," "I'm a good thinker," and "I'm sensitive and caring," may all represent preferred attributions of self. People also may have preferred explanations for actions they take.

For example, "I did X because I love my child," or "I did Y because I would do anything for a friend," might constitute preferred explanations. On the other hand, the thought that "I did X to be manipulative or controlling," might violate a person's preference. In general, we regard "preferred view" as a narrative concept—a fluid, evolving set of ideas about the self that embraces past, present, and future dimensions. Preferred views are inferred by the stories people tell about their lives.

Gleaning a person's preferred view can be a slippery business.

There is no simple, direct route, such as asking, "How do you prefer to be seen by others?" or "What is your preferred view, anyway?" that yields a clear and accurate answer. Furthermore, although we may react emotionally when we don't act as we'd like or when we feel that others don't see us as we want them to, we may not be clear about our wishes and intentions. Even when we are clear, we don't often articulate our preferences to others. We rarely say things such as, "You know, I prefer to be seen as a brilliant therapist. That's why my vein popped when you questioned my approach to helping that client."

Preferred views of self are inferred by asking a host of preference questions. For example, we asked Jean's father how he felt when he lost his temper. Did he feel good about himself or bad about himself? We also inquired about how he thought his wife regarded his interactions with Jean, and whether her response to him was preferred or not. We asked how he felt about earlier times in his relationship with Jean, when things were going better. And, we inquired about current aspects of his life such as his work as a teacher. Did he enjoy teaching? How did he think his students and coworkers regarded him? We also asked how he felt about how his own parents dealt with him as a teenager. Was he acting like his father acted? Did he prefer to act like his father?

Out of this inquiry, we gleaned that Jean's father preferred to see himself as a good teacher and a caring and involved father. It mattered a great deal to him that he was respected and that his advice was valued. He didn't like himself when he lost control of his temper, and he wasn't at all happy with how he thought his wife regarded him. He wanted to be different from his own father but was beginning to wonder whether he was. He was most comfortable with his son's view of him. John was the only member of the family who he felt regarded him with respect, who saw him as he wanted to be seen. Conversations with Jean revealed that she preferred to be seen as smart, capable, competent, and independent. She was pretty sure that her father did not see her in these ways. These discrepancies in viewpoint bring us to our next assumption about problem evolution.

Assumption 4. People experience negative and unsettling emotions such as frustration, sadness, and anxiety when (1) they behave in ways that are discrepant with preferred views of self, (2) they see themselves in ways that are discrepant with preferred views, and (3) they imagine that others see them in ways that are discrepant with preferred views.

An assumption of Carl Rogers's client-centered therapy was that people experienced unsettling emotions when there was a gap between their ideal self and their actual self, or self as perceived. Effective therapy occurred when the therapist assumed a critical position or stance that helped the client to experience "unconditional positive regard." Thus, the client's view of the therapist's view of her was seen as key to closing the troublesome gap between ideal self and self as perceived. Rogers was an individual therapist who focused on internal conflicts. Although Rogers described how "conditional positive regard" of parents and influential adults affected children's emotional development and shaped problems, he didn't involve parents or family members in the actual therapy (Rogers, 1951).

The work of R. D. Laing and his colleagues (Laing et al., 1966) added what we call a "cognitive-interactional" dimension. Although Laing never touched on the concept of preferred view, one of his most important, yet neglected, contributions to the field of family therapy was the notion of "disjunctive attributions." Laing wrote eloquently about the pain people experience when they perceive a gap between their own intentions and the attributions others assign to their motives. He said that "there is a strong tendency to feel guilt, anxiety, anger or doubt, if self attributions are disjunctive with attributions made about the self by other" (p. 152). According to Laing, disjunctive attributions are experienced from three vantage points. These include one's view of self, one's view of the other, and one's view of the other's view of self. When one's view of self grows out of sync with one's view of the other and with one's view of the other's view of self, emotional distress results. To Laing (1970), people experienced these gaps as internal "knots" that, on occasion, literally drove them crazy. One of Laing's most poignant portrayals of this process appeared in an evocative book called *The Divided Self*, which depicted the dark descent into schizophrenic thinking spurred on by the entangling web of disjunctive knots (Laing, 1960). What Laing described experientially as a "knot," we portray graphically in a problem cycle.

In describing our approach, we will use the term "disjunction" or "disjunctive attributions" to refer to the gap between how people *prefer* to be seen by others and how they see others seeing them. The experience of disjunction supplies the fuel that gets problem cycles going and keeps them going. We will consider how problems evolve as this gap widens and how problems resolve as this gap narrows. In this sense our definition of the concept of "disjunction" combines the individual–experiential contributions of Rogers with the interactional–experiential contributions of Laing to portray how people become stuck in their socially constructed predicaments.

Laing suggested that people experience disjunctive attributions, as if tied up in twisted knots that they can't loosen. The painful experi-

ence of disjunction was also described quite eloquently by William
James (1890/1984) many years ago:

> Those images in the minds of other men are, it is true, things outside of
> me, whose changes I perceive just as I perceive any other outward
> change. But the pride and shame which I feel are not concerned merely
> with those changes. I feel as if something else had changed too, when I
> perceived my image in your mind to have changed for the worse, some-
> thing in me to which that image belongs, and which a moment ago I felt
> inside of me, big and strong and lusty, but now weak, contracted and col-
> lapsed. (p. 97)

The emotional effects of disjunctive attributions brings us to our next
assumption about problem construction.

*Assumption 5. Problematic interactions often emerge as one or
more people begin to see others seeing them in ways discrepant with
how they prefer to be seen. This often happens at times of family transition, when views of self and other are changing, fluid, and unsettled.*

Events that occur during times of transition in families are significant to problem construction, because they awaken a search for new
meaning. At these times of flux, family members may begin to reconsider how they are seen by others close to them. The idea that relationships change when people notice something different about important
others was discussed in depth by Gregory Bateson (1988). According
to Bateson, shifts in interactional patterns occur when people respond
to "news of difference" (p. 28). What may seem at first glance to be an
ordinary event, such as eating popcorn in the living room, staying out
beyond a curfew, choosing a new friend who rides motorcycles and
sports tattoos, or not coming home on time for dinner, supply the raw
material for problem formation. If an event construed as "different"
challenges how people prefer to be seen and alters how they think others see them, new action is likely to emerge. This new behavior may
set in motion problematic interactions.

Ironically, there are many occasions in which what may appear to
be a more grievous or upsetting event, such as the onset of major illness, may *not* lead to problems beyond the illness itself. A person may
draw on existing strengths to "tough the illness out," or "not give in to
it," so that intimate others continue to perceive the person as unchanged. The person's preferred view in this sense remains intact, un-
shaken by the event and the ensuing actions of others, so that the idea
of a problem (beyond the upsetting event itself) never materializes.
Life is actually filled with such nonproblem scenarios, although we
tend not to notice them.

This assumption about problem evolution expands upon a basic premise of the MRI model mentioned earlier, that problems develop from the mishandling of ordinary life difficulties. From this perspective, people "slip into" problem-maintaining patterns more by accident than by structural or systemic design. Jeffrey Bogdan (1986) referred to this process as "accidentalism" (p. 35) to convey the random, not entirely predictable path to problems in the MRI approach. Steve de Shazer (1985) touched on a similar theme in describing how problems evolve out of "damned bad luck" (p. 18). A seemingly trivial event can trigger the onset of a major problem by jostling the preexisting views of those affected by the event. Whether a life event or an "accident" turns into an enduring problem hinges not only on how the event is construed but also on whether disjunctive views of self and other emerge in the wake of the event. Although events that we can't control or predict happen in life, there is some predictability as to whether problems develop. If an event challenges a person's preferred view and alters how he or she sees others seeing him or her, there is an increased probability that problems will develop. Beyond randomness, there is method to this process of problem construction.

In order to understand how transitional events affect problems, it's essential to know something about life before the event. When the conversation with Jean and her family turned to the preproblem past, more clues to the mystery of problem construction were found. The following conversation took place between the therapist and Jean, with her brother present.

LUND: Was there a time when you believed your dad thought well of you?

JEAN: He used to think I was smart.

LUND: When was that?

JEAN: A few years ago.

LUND: What were you two doing differently then?

JEAN: He used to take me skiing.

LUND: I don't think I get it. How did that indicate that he thought you were smart?

JEAN: Because he taught me to ski, and I learned so fast that he used to joke about it to his friends.

LUND: How was that for you?

JEAN: That was fun. We did it with golf, too.

LUND: You did what with golf?

JEAN: He taught me. I did good . . . he would tease his friends about how I was going to beat them all before I left junior high school.

LUND: Do you still do things together?

JEAN: No.

LUND: What happened?

JEAN: I don't know . . . he just got mean . . . (*tears*).

LUND: Do you think Dad thinks you are at all smart now?

JEAN: No . . . I thought he would be happy that I got good grades in school.

LUND: He's not?

JEAN: All he does is question how I get such good grades when I can't remember to do things that he asks at home . . . I can't stand him anymore.

LUND: Would you mind if I asked your dad about the skiing and golf and told him what you told me about that? I would really like to know how that was for him.

JEAN: That's fine with me.

This conversation revealed how Jean interpreted the changes in her relationship with her father over time. She used to feel good when her father saw her as "smart," but she thinks he no longer does. She expresses sadness about this gap between how she'd prefer to be seen and how she now imagines that her father thinks of her. She also speaks about her preferences. She prefers not to be fighting with her father, and recalls longingly the times when they were close, when he taught her skiing and complimented her to his friends. All this would be news to Dad, who hadn't the faintest idea that his daughter respected him or valued his input. Once upon a time, Jean's father experienced his daughter's love, trust, respect, and admiration. The typical adolescent transition of growing up and away from parents was made more painful by his perception that Jean lost all semblance of love and respect for him.

The intensity of Jean's apparent movement away from her father was fueled by disjunctive attributions, by her assumption that her father regarded her in a negative light. She was furious that her father saw her as "stupid" and incompetent, and she entertained little hope that her father would ever see her as she preferred. The effect on current behavior was that Jean refused to go along with her father's requests and would never apologize for forgetting about a family rule, as her brother did. The more convinced Jean became that her father thought her to be stupid, incompetent, and unworthy of his respect, the more she wore her defiance like a badge, concealing her preference for closeness and masking her sadness with sarcasm and anger.

The conversation with Jean's parents went as follows:

LUND: I enjoyed talking with your children. Jean was telling me about some fun that you and she had.

MR. RYAN: (*looking confused*) She told you about us having fun?

LUND: I was a bit surprised myself . . . she mentioned that you taught her to ski and golf and that she had the sense that you enjoyed it, too . . . she seemed pleased that you enjoyed it.

MR. RYAN: That's what you talked about?

LUND: That was part of what we talked about . . . do you folks talk much about that?

MR. RYAN: (*Mrs. Ryan smiling and looking on*) No, I'm very surprised she brought that up. I thought she forgot anything I did that might be good . . . how did that come up?

LUND: I was asking her about when things were going well . . . can I ask you both the same thing?

MR. RYAN: Well, I guess I would have to agree with Jean for a change. Things were very good then.

LUND: What made them good for you?

MR. RYAN: She was interested in what I had to say.

LUND: You mean she cooperated?

MR. RYAN: Pretty much. She was always a bit challenging.

LUND: I don't think I understood what you just said about her interest in what you had to say.

MRS. RYAN: I think what he means is that she used to show more interest in her father and want to learn about things he did.

LUND: Is that accurate?

MR. RYAN: Yeah, I think so . . . she doesn't seem to care for me or anything about me.

LUND: How is that for you?

MR. RYAN: It hurts.

LUND: When did things change?

MR. RYAN: When she went to her new school, made some new friends, and had no interest in spending time with the family.

MRS. RYAN: She spent less time with her dad and used the wise guy humor that he had taught her on him . . . he didn't like it.

Mr. Ryan seemed surprised that Jean might have anything good to say about him, or that she might speak of occasions in which she saw him as he wished. He, too, expressed hurt about the changes in their relationship. He and his wife recalled with nostalgia the times when Jean showed an interest in what he had to say. As Jean approached adolescence, went to a new school, and made new friends, she *acted as if* she didn't respect her father's advice anymore. Her father's temper outbursts were an outgrowth of the experience of disjunction. The more convinced he became that his daughter found him unworthy of regard, the more he attempted to command her respect through force. His preference for closeness and for being a helpful guide in Jean's quest for independence were no longer visible to Jean.

Jay Efran and his colleagues (1988) said, "Objectivist therapists want to know what *really* happened in the past; constructivist therapists are more interested in 'history' as a key to the unfolding family narrative that gives contemporary events their meaning" (p. 28). It's important to understand how past stories or narratives of people's lives help give meaning to events in the present. These stories affect how people view "news of difference" in relationships. As Mr. Ryan looked back, he remembered his own troubled adolescence. He recalled constant arguing with his father, who never understood him and died before they had a chance to resolve their conflicts. He vowed to do things differently and remain close to his daughter. Mr. Ryan perceived changes in Jean as she became an adolescent. He interpreted these changes to mean that she was moving away from him, a worrisome construction shaped by this past narrative. Mrs. Ryan's story of her own adolescence was similar to Jean's. Although she too had conflicts with her parents, they resolved as family members negotiated this challenging life transition. Mrs. Ryan viewed Jean's new and different adolescent behavior as "normal," a nonproblematic construction shaped by her past narrative.

Thus, what emerged from conversations with Jean and her family was a story of misunderstanding and conflict emerging during a time of family transition. As Jean reached adolescence, she showed more interest in friends. As she grew more independent, she appeared to disregard her parents' input. Jean's mother took these developments in stride. As she noticed news of difference, she perceived no challenge to her preferred view. Jean's father, on the other hand, felt threatened. He questioned whether these changes meant that Jean no longer loved or needed him. This unsettling view of self in the eyes of an important other propelled problem-maintaining behavior into motion.

Assumption 6. As problem cycles evolve, views of self and other become more fixed and actions more restricted. Repetitions of the cycle reinforce disjunctive attributions, escalate negative emotions, and promote more-of-the-same behavior.

As Mr. Ryan increased his efforts to give "input" to Jean in ways that undermined her sense of independence, she grew more defiant. He began to feel his daughter shunning him, which heightened his hurt, then anger, and fueled his futile attempts to command respect. The more upset and critical he became toward Jean, the more Mrs. Ryan acted in ways that suggested that she, too, disrespected him. Now he felt his wife regarded him in ways discrepant with his preferred view.

As the gap widened between how Mr. Ryan preferred to be seen and how he saw others seeing him, his distress and volatile behavior increased. He failed to notice occasions in which Jean treated him as he wished. Memories of Jean's respect for him, of skiing lessons and other happy times, faded. It was hard to imagine a future in which Mr. Ryan might once again be an important part of his daughter's life.

Disjunctive attributions also limited the range of behavior shown by Jean and her mother. Mrs. Ryan preferred to see herself as a competent mother and a loving wife, yet she felt that she couldn't get through to her daughter or her husband to stop their ugly arguing. Her failure to help caused her to doubt her own virtues as partner and parent. Shuttle diplomacy became Mother's only hope to remedy an increasingly hopeless situation. Meanwhile, the more coercive and critical Dad became, and the more conciliatory Mom became, the less Jean gave an inch. She refused to apologize even to her mother for misdeeds and stopped asking either parent for assistance in any way that might indicate to them that they mattered, even just a little.

The problem evolved into something fixed and static. It became a real "thing" that everyone noticed and that organized day-to-day life of the family. This "thingification" of the problem captures our final assumption about problem construction.

Assumption 7. As problematic interaction comes to dominate family life, family members become more convinced that a problem really exists and locate its cause in perceived deficiencies of self and other.

INTEGRATING STRATEGIC AND NARRATIVE CONCEPTS

In the 1970s and 1980s, strategic therapists maintained a narrow focus on immediate interaction and downplayed the importance of people's constructions about the past and future. Narrative therapists added the broad sweep of time to our understanding of human predicaments. Understanding how the broad narrative landscape shapes the narrow immediate situation, and how the narrow immediate situation shapes the broad narrative landscape is integral to understanding problem construction and problem deconstruction.

Cloé Madanes, a leader in the development of the strategic approach, describes therapy in a way that captures this integration of past, present, and future. Note her emphasis on narrative in this passage from her book *Sex, Love and Violence* (Madanes, 1990):

> If a therapist must have a theory of personality, then the most helpful one is that of an identity as a mental, abridged anthology of stories, any one of which can be replaced by a story from the total collection. Therapy thus involves editing the abridged edtion of perceptions of the present and past. A change in these perceptions is a change in the personality, and a change of shared perceptions is a change in the relationship. (p. 247)

Stories from the past, whether they are told or not, influence the development and maintenance of present interaction in ways that may not be known to the current protagonists. Unbeknownst to Jean, her mother and father looked back on their own adolescences with very different perspectives. Mr. Ryan's story of his relationship with his own father and how this changed for the worse as he approached adolescence is relevant to his present "framing" of Jean's behavior. Similarly, Mrs. Ryan's story of her "normal" relationship with her mother during adolescence, and her sense that things went well during that transition, fits with her present "framing" of her daughter's behavior. Past narrative accounts affect how transitional events are interpreted and shape how people respond to "news of difference."

When problematic interaction comes to dominate family life, the lens through which people view self and other narrows. Certain features of the broad narrative landscape are not noticed, whereas those that are emphasized reinforce negative feelings. Present actions that might indicate that Jean respects her father are not noticed by him. Current behaviors that might imply that Mr. Ryan thinks well of his daughter are overlooked by her. Similarly, preferred stories from the past are forgotten or recast in light of current negative views. While embroiled in problematic interactions, people don't see a preproblem past, don't notice current exceptions to problems, and don't envision a future without the problem.

The integration of narrative and strategic concepts brings together past, present, and future dimensions of individual and family life. Psychotherapists tend to emphasize one to the exclusion of the other, which obscures the exquisite interplay of time. For example, psychodynamic therapists often criticize behavior therapists and strategic family therapists for focusing only on here-and-now symptoms and ignoring their roots. Here-and-now therapies are regarded as "not deep enough." Similarly, present-oriented therapists, who emphasize brevity and practicality, are often intolerant of detours into the past. By linking narrative and strategic concepts, we suggest that key stories from the past inform the present predicament, which in turn informs how people recall their pasts and envision their futures. By understanding the process of problem construction in terms of all three time dimensions, we're better able to select key stories to talk about in therapy that will alter the present predicament, as well as reorient people to their pasts and futures.

THE SELF AND THE SYSTEM

Our understanding of problem construction takes into account how individuals come to view self and other, and how these views affect what they do. In this way, meaning and action are inextricably linked. By adding the dimension of viewing to a problem-cycle formulation, we are taking a step toward the self-system integration called for in Gregory Bateson's book *Steps to an Ecology of Mind* (Bateson, 1972). We are locating an inner circle of meaning within an outer circle of behavioral interaction that maintains problems. The importance of understanding each individual's construction of his or her situation at the "self" level is persuasively stated by Michael Nichols (1987). He reminds us that ultimately, it is individuals who think, feel, and act—and who initiate changes in systems.

> Constructive change occurs when individual family members develop new perspectives that lead them to new actions. Therefore, therapeutic intervention must reach and motivate individuals. Because the actions of family members are coordinated in patterned interactions, therapists can sometimes effect change while thinking in terms of interaction, of process instead of persons. Even then, however, the interventions succeed or fail to the extent that they mobilize persons to think and act differently. (p. 38)

An understanding of how individuals construct problematic views of self and other is relevant to finding the path to their deconstruction.

Although we'll describe in more detail the steps to problem resolution in Chapters 6 and 7, let's review briefly what happened with Jean and her family. For this family, our inquiry into the preproblem past revealed stories of preference. When Jean spoke longingly about skiing and playing golf with her father, she unveiled an alternative view about her father that he had long since forgotten. We learned that she really did respect him as a teacher, particularly when she felt supported and complimented by him. In fact, her sadness about losing closeness with him, along with losing confidence in his positive view of her, explained her current defiance. We now had something new and different to offer Mr. Ryan about what Jean was up to.

The disclosure of this "hidden narrative" prompted a rapid change in her father's behavior. After hearing about Jean's reminiscences and preferences, Mr. Ryan casually mentioned to Jean how he used to enjoy skiing and playing golf with her. He said this positively, matter-of-factly, refraining from adding unnecessary editorial comments about how "unenjoyable" she was to be with now. Although Jean didn't warm immediately to this remembrance, she later responded by asking something of her father that might appear at first glance to be ordinary, but represented a major departure from their usual pattern. She asked her father to help her with a difficult homework assignment. Although Mr. Ryan didn't see this event as monumental, he was surprised and pleased. The therapist took the opportunity to frame Jean's request as another demonstration of how she "really" viewed her father. The idea that his daughter still respected him as a teacher introduced hope. This enabled Mr. Ryan to envision future solutions.

The conversation with Jean's parents about their own adolescences set the stage for change. The therapist supported Mrs. Ryan's frame for understanding Jean's defiant behavior, suggesting that this was ordinary adolescent unpleasantness rather than a concerted campaign to distance from an unneeded father. As Mr. Ryan reflected on his own adolescence and reconsidered where Jean might be coming from, he began to see that his extrapolations from his own negative experience didn't necessarily fit for Jean. After all, unlike his own relationship with his father, Mr. Ryan's relationship with his daughter was very close at one time. He began to explain Jean's defiance differently. Perhaps she felt compelled to prove that she could be independent because she felt so close to her father during her childhood. Perhaps defiance was spurred on by *his* criticism. The experience of criticism inspired Jean to show her father that she didn't need his damned teaching anymore. After all, she was a lot like him—stubborn, proud, unyielding. By asking her father for help with homework, Jean showed him how he was still a teacher in her eyes, supporting a preferred explanation for the evolution of defiance. With this, Mr. Ryan altered his approach. He softened.

Over the course of eight visits with family members in various combinations, Jean and her father began joking with each other once again. They spent more time together, although much less than during Jean's preadolescence. Yet, it was enough time for Mr. Ryan to become reacquainted with his importance to his daughter and for the two to reclaim a loving relationship. Jean's mother was delighted that the "ugly arguing" stopped. She felt free to have a relationship with her husband and daughter without being pressured to take sides.

By making story selection more precise, therapy can be brief, practical, and efficient. Brevity and practicality aren't necessarily enhanced by focusing only on here-and-now patterns of behavior. Drawing out key stories from the past that alter how people see self and other in the present can produce swift results. Once Mr. Ryan learned that Jean recalled the past with longing and sadness, he reconsidered his present approach and made rapid and impactful changes. In this sense, the *poetic* possibilities in the narrative approach (drawing out preferred reminiscences and stories) weave nicely with the strategic emphasis on the *practical*.

In this chapter we presented a theory of problem construction that integrates concepts from strategic and narrative family therapy and from individual and family therapy. The assumptions we make about how people construct problems have clear implications for how to converse with people in helpful ways. In the next two chapters, we explore in more detail how to conduct a therapeutic conversation— how to start it, develop it, and conclude it. We begin our discussion of the therapeutic conversation with the first phone call, when we decide whom to see.

—5—

The Strategy of Conversation, Part I: Approaching the Therapeutic Conversation

A therapeutic conversation begins with the first phone call. This is when we arrange the first appointment and decide whom to see. It's also our first contact with the person defining the problem, and it presents an opportunity to connect with that person's preferences and positive intentions.

THE FIRST PHONE CALL

In this conversation, we elicit the caller's views about being in therapy. We find out how the caller arrived at the decision to make an appointment. Was it of his or her own or someone else's urging? If someone persuaded the person to call, how did he or she feel about this advice? Is the caller calling out of coercion or strong personal conviction? We also find out how important others view this decision to seek professional help. Do other family members know about the caller's decision to seek help? Whether consulted or not, how do they feel about the idea of therapy? Would they like to participate at some point? How does the caller feel about others joining him or her for the first session? Would he or she prefer that we consult other family members? These are the kinds of questions we ask over the telephone. The answers we get determine whom we see initially and whom we talk with later.

Since we have no preconceived notion that all family members should be seen together or that one individual is the "real" patient and must be seen immediately, we usually go along with the caller's preference about whom to see. In fact, the first phone call presents an opportunity to show interest in people's hopes, intentions, and experiences.

Consider this example of a telephone conversation in which Joe arranged an appointment with Sylvia, a 40-year-old woman who was troubled about her 15-year marriage to her husband, Harry.

SETTING AN APPOINTMENT WITH SYLVIA

When Sylvia Walker called for a consultation, she sounded nervous. She said that the appointment would be for herself, but she wanted to discuss her marriage. Joe asked Sylvia if her husband knew she was calling. Sylvia said that Harry didn't know, and that she didn't want him to know. "Why not?" Joe asked. Sylvia said that Harry had a bad temper. "Did Harry's temper have anything to do with your decision to come in alone?" Joe wondered. "Not really," Sylvia said. "If Harry comes in, he'll just make things more difficult for me. I just need to talk some things over. And please don't tell me to leave him. That's what everyone says."

The therapist wondered what Sylvia meant about Harry's temper and was curious about her statement that others advised her to leave Harry. Was Harry prone to violence? Was Sylvia worried about her safety? Was that why she kept her decision to make an appointment a secret from Harry? Joe asked, "Did Harry's temper have anything to do with your decision not to tell him about your appointment? Were you concerned that you'd be in any danger if you mentioned meeting with me?" Sylvia assured Joe that she wasn't afraid for her safety. She simply didn't want to engage in a conversation with Harry about the marriage until she was clear as to how she wanted to talk with him. She didn't want Harry's predictable negativity about therapy to dictate her decision about what to do. She preferred to talk with a professional who'd be "objective," not to friends and family who weren't.

By eliciting Sylvia's wishes regarding participation in therapy, it became clear whom to see first. The therapist also obtained information to build on. He learned about Sylvia's commitment to make an independent decision about her marriage and not succumb to the influence of Harry's temper. Joe began to compose a picture of how Sylvia preferred to be seen as a person, which would be helpful in planning future conversations with her and other family members. Sylvia also offered some clues about how she viewed Harry and how she thought Harry viewed therapy. These clues might prove helpful in figuring out how to talk with Harry if and when it made sense to meet with him.

THE PRINCIPLE OF GENERATIVE CONVERSATION

The question of whom to see in therapy and when to see them is governed by the broader question of what conversations are most helpful in solving problems. We hope that conversations between the therapist and one or more family members in the room are only the starting point to future helpful conversations between parents and children, husbands and wives, children and their friends, parents and school officials, and others that take place outside the treatment room.

As an example, consider the conversation Sylvia had with Harry outside the therapy room. Joe and Sylvia met three times before she decided to talk with Harry about the marriage and his participation in therapy. In these three meetings, Joe and Sylvia explored Sylvia's views of the marriage and how these views changed over time. They examined past conversations between Sylvia and Harry about difficulties in the relationship. They discussed how these past conversations affected Sylvia's thoughts and feelings about herself, her view of Harry, and her confidence in the marriage. Joe and Sylvia speculated about how these conversations affected Harry's behavior, Harry's thoughts and feelings about himself, and Harry's views of Sylvia and the marriage. They discussed occasions in which Sylvia felt conversations went well and when they didn't.

During these three individual sessions, Sylvia gained clarity about what direction she wanted the marriage to head. She felt she "thought things through" well enough to talk with Harry about her concerns. Sylvia's conversation with Harry outside the treatment room became a turning point in the process of change.

In this transforming conversation, Sylvia spoke clearly with Harry about the marriage she wanted to have. She took an unequivocal position against temper outbursts. She said she hated it when Harry criticized her and called her names, and when he acted this way with the children. She also didn't like it when Harry cursed when he couldn't find things or couldn't repair a household item he was trying to fix. She worried that Harry's angry self-derogatory remarks would be followed by his putting his fist through a wall or door, while screaming at the top of his lungs. It didn't matter, she said, that Harry never struck her or the children. His temper outbursts frightened her and the children and caused them to withdraw from a man they loved. This was not the family environment Sylvia wanted. She said that if things stayed this way, she might leave Harry.

Sylvia's conversational approach was assertive, nonblaming, respectful, and compassionate. She set the tone for the kind of marriage she wanted and shifted the responsibility to Harry to decide whether his preferred picture of the marriage dovetailed with hers. After Sylvia engaged in this pivotal conversation with Harry outside the treatment room, Harry decided to call to make his own appointment.

With Harry's phone call, the problem definition changed. The problem became Harry's temper rather than Sylvia's confusion about her marriage. At this stage in the therapeutic conversation, the burden for deciding about the marriage transferred to Harry, who was now the one expressing anxiety about where the marriage was heading. When Harry met with Joe, he seemed motivated to prove to Sylvia that he could control his temper, and that she could count on him to be a supportive husband. Change was occurring in Sylvia and Harry's marriage, even though the therapist hadn't talked with them together in the room.

Family therapists sometimes worry that seeing one member of a family reinforces the linear notion that one person is the real problem. Certainly, if managed poorly, individual conversations may set up the perception that the therapist has an alliance with one spouse against the other. Parents might experience the therapist as being on the child's side, and not theirs. Or a father might think the therapist is on the mother's side, and not his. A well-managed conversation with people separately, however, fosters alliances with individuals without creating coalitions against other family members.

Consider, for example, what might have happened if the therapist, as an expert in couple therapy, conveyed to Sylvia Walker over the telephone that he only met with couples together. Would Sylvia have gone elsewhere, since this particular therapist didn't do what she preferred? Or, would she have complied with the therapist and assumed that since *he* was the expert, she should depend on his advice? Such compliance could have affected Sylvia's position in the ongoing therapy, rendering her a more passive listener than an active participant. Would this insistence on seeing the couple together, made by a male therapist, mirror existing relationship patterns in the marriage? In Sylvia's mind, would the therapist become yet another man who, like her husband, considered Sylvia's preferences unimportant? Sylvia's decision to make up her own mind about her marriage was a unique event that fit within her preferred picture of a future marriage in which she had a stronger voice. The therapist, inadvertently, could have silenced Sylvia's voice by insisting that he see her and Harry together.

Many therapists prefer to meet with couples together. Often this decision is compatible with what clients want. Certainly, skilled couple therapists can conduct conjoint sessions in ways that encourage persons to express their views and be heard by their partners. Thus, new conversations may take place inside the treatment room that generalize outside the treatment room. Although we prefer to conduct some sessions individually with partners in a relationship to ensure that we understand each person's narrative account, we also meet with couples together. Typically, we arrange conjoint sessions to clarify the therapy contract, to consolidate progress, and to accommodate client preferences about format. The point we want to emphasize here is that therapists should be wary of *imposing* their preferences for conversational format on clients who have different wishes.

As Sylvia talked about her relationship with Harry from the vantage point of her own preferences and intentions, her thoughts about the problem changed. It was then that she decided to talk with Harry about her present and past concerns and her future aspirations. And it was through this *new conversation* that the problem was redefined. Therapists should remain alert to shifting problem definitions as therapy progresses and be prepared to talk with different people as the need arises. Change occurs through the process of generative conversation.

INTENTIONS AND EFFECTS

The conversations with Sylvia and Harry illustrate another theme in our approach—the relationship between intentions and effects. Helpful conversations invite people to take clear positions about their intentions, to consider the effects of their behavior on others, and to indicate whether these effects are preferred or not. Sylvia talked to Harry in a way that fit her preferred view of being a caring partner and mother, who was opposed to temper outbursts. She also articulated what kind of marriage she wanted. In this way, she invited Harry to take a clear position about his own behavior, its effects on others, and whether these effects were preferred. Harry was invited to say what kind of husband and father he'd like to be and what kind of marriage he'd like to be in. What if Harry said he was comfortable losing his temper and enjoyed the silencing effect his volatile behavior had on others? What if Harry's version of a preferred marriage was that *he* was in charge, and family members should respect him when he exploded? This position would signify that Harry was *not* a customer for therapy.

This brings us to a principle about the limits of helpful conversations. When people view their own actions and see the effects of their actions on themselves and on others as congruent with their intentions, there is *no problem* for them to work on in therapy. For example, Sylvia indicates that there's a problem because her intention is to have a close relationship with Harry. However, this preference is discrepant with her experience of the relationship. In spite of her efforts, Harry is not acting in a way that promotes warmth and connection. Sylvia doesn't feel her talks with Harry have had the desired effect. Thus, Sylvia defines a problem. For there to be a workable problem in therapy, there must be a gap between intentions and effects.

Therapists can help people talk with each other in respectful ways that *invite* nondefensive, nonblaming dialogue about preferences. Helpful conversations elicit preferences about intentions and effects. After engaging in a helpful conversation with Harry, Sylvia and Joe will learn about Harry's intentions. They'll find out whether Harry wants to have Sylvia and the children retreat from him. They'll soon know whether Harry would like to have a close or distant marriage, whether he likes or doesn't like losing his temper, whether his behavior fits with his intentions, and whether his actions yield the effects he desires. Should Sylvia engage in a helpful conversation with Harry, he will inform her about whether he's a customer for couple counseling and help her decide how to proceed. Although therapists can influence people to have helpful conversations with each other, they don't have control over the positions people take once these conversations occur.

Sylvia's telling Harry what she wants has the potential to raise Harry's anxiety and make him defensive. He may not hear what Sylvia has to say, much less define clearly what he thinks and feels. So how did Sylvia get around the usual querulous quarreling and inspire Harry to take a position that would resolve her own indecision about the marriage? The secret was that Sylvia avoided making statements that contradicted Harry's preferred view. She spoke with Harry in a way that was consistent with his being a competent, sensitive, loving husband. Harry didn't feel that he had to defend himself against accusations of being a bad husband or father. Instead, he was invited to clarify why a man Sylvia loved and respected would act in ways that promoted her distance.

The basis of Sylvia's helpful conversation with Harry was that she connected with his positive potential, while being interested in his preferences. She assumed the same position with her spouse that we encourage therapists to take with their clients as they begin therapeutic conversations. Because Sylvia approached Harry in this respectful way, there was no danger that Harry would experience Sylvia and the therapist siding against him. If anything, he'd perceive them as on his side and thus be interested in becoming part of the dialogue.

FROM JOINING TO CONNECTING WITH PREFERENCES

"Joining" is the term structural family therapists introduced that helped family therapists realize that they were part of the systems they were trying to change. Minuchin (1974) emphasized the importance of forming a relationship with each family member before attempting to confront or challenge problematic patterns of interaction. The concept of joining implied that there were individual selves living in larger systems, and that therapists needed to recognize each person's hopes, intentions, and preferences before attempting to rearrange their relationships with others.

The idea of joining steered family therapists away from thinking of systems as impersonal cybernetic machines that swallowed up individuals. Joining brought family therapists into the conversation as active participants. They moved closer to people, sitting forward in their chairs, warmly connecting with each person's uniqueness. Joining suggested that therapists could connect with people through the process of conversation.

Our approach to connecting with people is predicated on the concept of preferred view. Connecting with preferences not only forges an empathic link with people, but it also sets in motion the process of change. According to our assumptions about problem construction, problems evolve out of discrepancies between how people prefer to view themselves and how they think others regard them. Problems resolve as these troublesome gaps in perception narrow. The first step in promoting narrative solutions is for therapists to align with each person's preferred view. In this way, the therapist becomes one important other who regards the person in ways he or she would like. This invites people to talk about and consider how intimate others view them, and it opens up conversational opportunities inside and outside the treatment room. For example, in making the appointment with Sylvia Walker, Joe let Sylvia know that he respected her initiative. He let her know that he thought her ideas about therapy were important. This preference-promoting conversation set the stage for subsequent talks that would move toward problem resolution.

The idea of connecting with preferred views fits with a social constructionist perspective on empathy. We can empathize with each family member's experience of the problem without implying that anyone is right or wrong, that their actions are justified or not justified, or that their feelings are correct or incorrect. For example, we can empathize with Harry's experience of Sylvia's distance and his distress that she perceives him as unable to control his temper. This form of empathy challenges Harry to act in line with his own preference to be in control of his temper, and to convince Sylvia that she can trust him. Furthermore, our empathy with Harry in no way contradicts our empathy with Sylvia, who wants a loving marriage and prefers to live with a man who controls his temper. We can also empathize with Harry and Sylvia's shared pain that their marriage doesn't meet with their current expectations, and doesn't fit with their original reasons for choosing each other.

Let's consider another example of a preferred view confirming conversation with Stan, a 54-year-old man who suffered panic attacks intermittently for 30 years. After being problem free for 5 years, he had a full blown attack in his boss's office.

TALKING COMFORTABLY WITH A MAN
WHO HAS PANIC ATTACKS

Joe knew from Stan's family doctor, who made the referral, that Stan had a responsible position in his company, managing a department with 25 employees. Joe learned from Dr. Michaels that Stan called him after an embarrassing incident involving Stan's manager. Dr. Michaels let Joe know that it was difficult for Stan to make the appointment, and that he reluctantly agreed to call after some prodding.

Before meeting with Stan, Joe pondered how Stan might feel being responsible for managing 25 people and being urged to talk with a professional about anxiety he couldn't manage. Joe imagined that Stan would experience this contradiction as unsettling. He considered how to help Stan feel more "settled" before getting into the subject of his long-standing problem with panic.

After spending a few minutes listening to Stan's story about the recent panic attack in his boss's office, Joe decided to switch gears. Since the panic attack happened in his boss's office, and since Stan was a manager himself, Joe became curious about Stan's position in the company and his approach to management. The experience of having an attack in the presence of his boss seemed to contradict how Stan wished to be seen. He felt diminished, incompetent, powerless. The therapist didn't want to fix Stan's attention on this humiliating scene in the boss's office. He wanted to shift to other scenes and other offices.

Joe inquired about Stan's position in his company, where he worked, what he did, and who he was responsible for and to. Stan said he worked closely with his employees and went the extra yard to encourage and talk with them about their performance, whether good or bad. Joe then became curious about other areas of management in Stan's life. How did he manage relationships with his children and his now elderly parents? Stan described himself as a responsible man who often put others' needs before his own. Interestingly, Stan first began experiencing anxiety as he was helping his mother after she suffered her first heart attack. It was Stan, and not his younger siblings, who assumed the bulk of responsibility for visiting his mother on weekends, for talking to her doctor about her care, and relaying information back to his mother and father, who were both frightened. Another bout with panic attacks happened when Stan's ex-wife had a "nervous breakdown," and he took over all the responsibility for his children. In both instances, he concealed his symptoms from others and forged on with his caretaking duties, occasionally taking antianxiety medication so that he could still perform. It seemed that although Stan was an excellent manager of others, this often came at the expense of caring for himself.

As Joe spoke with Stan about his strengths as a manager of people, Stan perked up. He seemed less nervous, more animated, and eager to tell his story. These were signs that the therapist was on the right track, that he had connected with Stan's preferences and positive intentions. At that point, he steered the conversation over to how Stan managed himself. Joe asked Stan if he was as sensitive to his own discomfort as he was to the emotional needs of others. Thus, Joe and Stan entered a conversation about the problem of anxiety that was nondisjunctive, that fit with Stan's proven ability to be a caring manager. Joe then inquired further into the mystery of why panic attacks had returned to a place of prominence in Stan's life.

As you can see in this example, connecting with preferences isn't the same as cheerleading. The therapist didn't come out and say, "You're a fine manager," or "You're an in-control and competent guy." Nor did he make bold assertions like, "I bet if you can manage tough situations like that, you can find a way to manage your anxiety." Such comments are patronizing and suggest that therapists know more than clients know about who they "really" are and what they really can do. Connecting with preferences happens more subtly, by taking a sincere interest in the ordinary events of people's lives that reveal who they wish to be.

CREATING OPPORTUNITIES THROUGH HELPFUL CONVERSATIONS

The term "maneuverability" was used by strategic therapists to refer to ways of eliciting people's views that opened up options for prescriptive behavior change (Fisch et al., 1982). To the strategic therapist, maneuverability was about creating leverage, so that clients were more likely to follow a therapeutic directive.

The concept of maneuverability applies to our approach in the sense that we want to *stay flexible* in the therapeutic conversation and open opportunities for people to reconsider their actions and intentions. By connecting with preferred views, conversational latitude is enhanced in a number of ways. People give us valuable information about how they view themselves, as well as how they see important others in their past and present lives. They shift back and forth in time, relating key stories from the past that inform their current predicament, and offer up their preferred vision of the future. They talk more openly about their concerns. They begin to acknowledge the effects of their own actions on the maintenance of problems, and to consider doing things differently.

Whether therapists give people behavioral prescriptions or not, joining with preferred views also opens up conversations about new modes of action. People become more interested in talking with therapists about how to bring their own actions more into line with their preferences, which affords the therapist greater maneuverability in affecting behavior change. It's not imperative that therapists come up with clever task assignments or ingenious directives to get people to change. Rather, people get motivated to think of creative solutions on their own and talk them over with the therapist.

Finally, connecting with preferences allows therapists more room to make and recover from mistakes. We will give examples of bad moves and not-so-helpful conversations initiated by therapists that they are still able to rebound from and even use to advantage. When clients feel that therapists view them as competent, they are more forgiving. They usually give therapists a second chance to help them.

Let's now explore how therapists come across to clients when using this approach. What kind of ambience is created in the room? What's the client's experience of the therapist likely to be? What stance does a helpful therapist take in managing a helpful conversation?

THE COLUMBO POSITION

We prefer to use the image of the unassuming TV detective Columbo to capture the therapist's orientation in talking with people. This position combines a "not-knowing," humble curiosity with "knowing" how to decipher the patterns of conversation that produce impasses and how to help people get beyond the hurdles they call problems (see Anderson & Goolishian, 1992, for a discussion of the not-knowing position).

In the TV series, Lt. Columbo, played by Peter Falk, greeted suspects in his rumpled raincoat, asking questions in an interested, humble way. He usually invited people to help him and complimented them for their cooperation and astute observations. Although Columbo assumed a not-knowing position in asking curious questions, his know-how involved putting the pieces of the jigsaw puzzle together and arranging them into an order that explained or lent coherence to the various narrative accounts he elicited. With this, he solved the crime. And it was all done without excessive confrontation or bloodshed. Columbo came up with respectful solutions to crimes. It was as if suspects went off to jail with their "preferred views" intact. Whereas Columbo was disingenuous, that is, he knew all along who the culprit was, we are interested not in seeking the guilty party but in unraveling the mystery of how the problem evolved.

Helpful therapists are like good detectives in the Columbo tradition. They look for clues that reside in the tales people tell about their lives. They ask questions from a position of curiosity and respect, engaging help from people in putting together the puzzle of how their problem became a problem. The problem itself becomes a mystery that fails to represent the truth of who people really are, and commands an explanation. The therapeutic conversation is designed to unravel the mystery of how the problem evolved, so that new solutions emerge. The story of the problem, which is typically presented by the people affected by it as fixed, certain, and "known," becomes fluid and somewhat murky. Ultimately, the therapist cultivates a new explanation for the "mystery" of the problem that confirms people's preferences and helps them find solutions.

THE MYSTERY QUESTION

In keeping with this Columbo-like position, there is a key question that orients the therapeutic conversation. Sometimes, this question is posed directly to clients, whereas at other times therapists simply ask themselves the question, using it as a guide for further inquiry. We call this the mystery question, and it goes like this. How did someone with X preferred attributes (competent, in control, independent, etc.) wind up in Y situation (having depression, experiencing worry or fear, being watched over by others), and being viewed by others in Z ways (not competent or capable)?

Once we get to know how people wish to be seen by others, it's useful to enlist their help in explaining how they landed in their current fix, having a problem they don't want to have and being seen by others in ways they don't like. This mystery question opens an important discussion about the evolution of problems, which often offers clues to solutions. The question also encourages personal agency. People become interested in figuring out how they got into such a predicament and how to get themselves out of it. In this way, clients become active participants in mapping the path of the problem and generating solutions.

THE MAN WHO HAD PANIC ATTACKS (CONTINUED)

Let's return to Joe's conversation with Stan as an example of the effect of the mystery question. After inquiring about Stan's capabilities as a manager and discussing his talents in this area, Joe asked Stan why someone with such obvious sensitivity to others would have difficulty managing his own discomfort? This contradiction was puzzling, to say the least. Joe's curiosity about the management of self-comfort (in itself a reframing of the problem of anxiety), prompted Stan to recall two key stories.

In one (preferred) story, Stan offered an example of how he managed his discomfort with dentists by interviewing several dentists in the community. He finally found one who was sensitive to his fear about being confined to a dentist's chair. After revealing to the dentist how *he* wanted to be managed, Stan had no trouble getting through his first dental appointment without incident. Over the years, he gradually overcame his fear of dentists. This story contrasted with the story Stan told about his most recent panic attack. In this instance, Stan was poised to go on an important business trip, which involved a long drive. He had grown fearful of driving in rain or snow, and local weather forecasters predicted snow for his upcoming trip. This time, he concealed his apprehension from his boss and tried to talk himself into going on the trip, downplaying his anxiety as ridiculous. On the day of the trip, as he was finalizing plans with his boss, he had a severe panic attack in full view of his boss, who tried his best to comfort him and figure out what was wrong. When Stan finally revealed that he was dreading the long drive and the prospect of snow and ice, his boss calmly advised him to put off the trip until spring.

By the time Stan finished telling these two stories, it seemed that something had clicked. Mulling over the two vignettes, and comparing the outcomes, there was little doubt as to which outcome he preferred. Joe and Stan decided that the recent incident with his boss did not imply the return to a life of panic attacks, medication, and anxiety avoidance, as Stan had feared. Rather, it was a reminder that he lost sight of the solution to panic, which involved managing his own discomfort by helping others realize what *he* needed.

Left to ponder the mystery question, Stan rapidly came up with answers. He soon recognized that he already possessed the know-how to manage panic. He could simply apply the approach he took with the dentist and learn from his recent mismanagement of the business trip. After only three sessions, Stan felt confident that he could keep panic at bay in the future. Therapy ended with Stan feeling like a competent manager in many areas of his life, including his newfound executive approach to panic.

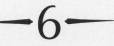

The Strategy of
Conversation, Part II:
Steps to Assessment

Let's walk through the steps taken in a therapeutic conversation with a 14-year-old girl named Rachel and her mother, Marion.

At the time we first met Rachel and her mother, Rachel was in a junior high special education class. Her grades were straight A's until fourth grade, at which point they started slipping. In the fifth and sixth grades, she started to fight with other girls at school and refused to comply with her teachers' requests. By seventh grade, the fighting at school was more pronounced, and at home Rachel began arguing with her mother and pulling away from her emotionally.

Shortly before our contact, Rachel and Marion attempted counseling but had a disappointing experience. After two sessions, Rachel expressed her displeasure to her mother. Marion encouraged Rachel to continue, but Rachel began disappearing before sessions. Rachel agreed to counseling again, only because her lawyer convinced her that it would look good to the court. Rachel was suspended from school after fighting with a classmate, then was found on school property taunting this same girl. The school principal lodged trespassing charges against her, and a court hearing was set to evaluate these charges. Because Rachel had been in so much trouble already—from talking back to teachers and fighting with other girls in school—the principal labeled her "incorrigible." Rachel's attorney told her that she could be placed in a special school, away from home.

STEPS TO HELPFUL CONVERSATIONS
(MAPPING THE EVOLVING PROBLEM)

Step 1. The therapist inquires about how the client got to the therapist's office. Was it of the person's own volition or someone else's urging? Did everyone involved agree with the advice to seek help, or did some feel forced to come in? Do family members have the same or different opinions about seeking professional help? How do these views reflect their personal preferences?

Step 2. The therapist elicits and accepts the client's definition of the problem.

The conversation with Rachel alone began as follows.

LUND: Your mother called and told me a little bit about why she wanted us to talk. Whose idea was it for you to come in?

RACHEL: I don't want nothing to do with it.

LUND: How did you end up here?

RACHEL: I came because my lawyer said I had to, for court.

LUND: The court ordered you to come?

RACHEL: No, my lawyer said if I came it would look good for next week. I don't know why.

LUND: What does your mom think of counseling?

RACHEL: She said it's up to me. If I want to help myself, I should go to counseling. I don't want to.

LUND: Why are you going to court?

RACHEL: I don't want to talk about it. Why don't you ask my mother?

LUND: You really don't want to be here, do you?

RACHEL: No.

The problem, as Rachel sees it, is that she has to go to court and therefore has to come for counseling to make a good impression on the judge. She also states that her mother has left it to her to decide about therapy. Neither mother nor daughter really prefers to see a therapist.

Step 3. The therapist asks whether the client has sought help before or been given advice about the present problem by others. Knowing how people have viewed other helpers gives a therapist important clues about how people prefer to be seen and how to join with them.

For Rachel, inquiring about other helpers was also helpful in fig-uring out what not to do.

LUND: Have you ever talked to a counselor?

RACHEL: One or two times.

LUND: How did it go?

RACHEL: I didn't want to talk to him, and he told me that I didn't know what I was talking about. He said I needed counseling, but I don't, and I didn't go back. I just want to get court over with and go back to school.

Rachel sheds some light on why she's not interested in talking with a counselor. Her past experience was that professionals spoke with her in ways that challenged her preferred view and fueled her resistance. If Tom attempts to persuade Rachel to talk to him or convince her that he could be helpful, Rachel might see him seeing her as not knowing what she is doing, and she will be less likely to talk.

Should Rachel chose not to speak with Tom, he might feel that Rachel sees him in a way that contradicts his own preferred view. He may then try harder to encourage Rachel to open up. This becomes a downhill conversational pattern. As you'll see, Tom accepts and re-spects Rachel's viewpoint about helpers, and the conversation moves along with little urging.

Step 4. Next, we consider the client's goals or preferred vision of the future. How would life be different if the "problem" went away?

In this case, the problem for Rachel is that various adults think she doesn't know what she is doing, is out of control, and needs to be in a special class or even in a residential placement. The therapist in-vites Rachel to express her own ideas about what's best for her.

LUND: You seem to think going back to school is best?

RACHEL: Yes.

LUND: You like it there?

RACHEL: I don't like the classes I'm in, but I want to go back to school and get in a regular class.

LUND: If the court decided on another placement, they'd probably arrange for something where adults are watching you even clos-er.

RACHEL: That's what I hate. I just want to go back to the regular class-es. I never get to see any of my friends now.

LUND: You seem pretty clear about what would be best for you. You just want to go back to regular classes.

Rachel moves from not being at all interested in talking to a therapist, to talking with some interest about her predicament. Simply being cu-rious about a person's views and not passing judgement on their rightness or wrongness can elicit a lot of useful information about problem development.

The therapist goes beyond neutrality (or passive acceptance of Rachel's views) when he says to Rachel, "You seem to know what's best for you." This is an example of connecting with her preferred view. Seeing Rachel as a competent, capable person who knows what's best for her runs counter to the prevailing idea that she needs to be watched closely by adults. Once Rachel sees the therapist seeing her in preferred ways, she'll become even more communicative. She'll speak more freely about how others think of and act toward her, and how she responds to their perceptions and actions.

Step 5. Inquire about how the client regards others, and how the client sees others seeing them.

LUND: What does your mom think of all this?

RACHEL: She thinks I don't know what I'm doing. She thinks I'm dumb.

LUND: She says that?

RACHEL: Well, she doesn't come right out and say it, but I know.

LUND: You can tell somehow?

RACHEL: She tells everybody that I don't know what I'm doing. She tells my sister, my aunt . . . everybody knows my business.

LUND: That doesn't sound so good.

RACHEL: It isn't.

LUND: You don't like everybody knowing your business?

RACHEL: (*with an angry tone*) No, I don't tell her nothing. I don't tell no-body nothing.

Step 6. As therapists ask about people's views, they also ask about their actions. Inquiries about viewing and doing go together.

LUND: If you talk to Mom, she tells everybody your business. If you talk to a counselor, they'll tell you you don't know what you're doing. I think I'm getting a pretty good idea why you don't want to talk to anyone.

RACHEL: If I get suspended, my mother tells my sister, my grandmother, everybody.

LUND: Does Mom talk with you about these things?

RACHEL: No.

LUND: So if things don't go well at school, Mom doesn't talk to you about it.

RACHEL: No. She just grounds me.

LUND: For how long?

RACHEL: I don't know. I know I'm grounded.

LUND: For how long now?

RACHEL: For 2 weeks so far, but I don't know when it ends.

LUND: Oh, I see. It's your basic endless grounding. Your mother doesn't say anything?

RACHEL: She says that if I keep it up, teachers and everybody will do something. I don't care. If someone bothers me, I'm not putting up with it.

LUND: What do you do when someone bothers you?

RACHEL: I fight back.

LUND: Are there a lot of bothersome people at that school?

RACHEL: Only a few, but they think they're tough, and teachers don't do anything. So I will.

LUND: Is that how this court thing came up?

RACHEL: Yes. Someone bothered a friend of mine—I straightened her out and the teacher got mad at me. The other girl got nothing.

LUND: How did you straighten her out?

RACHEL: I punched her in the face.

LUND: Then what happened?

RACHEL: I got suspended, but she threatened my friend again, so I went back to school. Then they said I was trespassing on school property, so I have to go to court.

LUND: What did your mom do?

RACHEL: She says she don't know what they will do, and I better listen to my lawyer, and go to counseling. I listened to my lawyer but I'm not going to counseling after court.

In the last two segments of conversation we learn that Rachel sees her mother seeing her as "dumb" and "not knowing what she's doing." Rachel also seems concerned that her sister, aunt, and grandmother may be developing this same view. Adding further to her distress, Rachel describes how her teacher sees her as not handling her conflicts, to the point that she gets suspended from school, whereas the girl who picked on her friend goes unpunished.

As people begin to talk about how others see them and act toward them, they often, without being asked, start to describe what they do to compensate for these unsettling views and actions. Rachel tries to assert her independence and rectify the unfairness that surrounds her by taking matters into her own hands. Unfortunately, this has the effect of further reprimand from school officials and even more vigilance by adults. Marion's "endless restriction" approach seems an attempt to pull in the reins on Rachel and take charge of her misbehavior, but it is ill-fated. Rachel sees her mom as tattling to relatives about her bad behavior while acting uncertain about what to do herself, and relinquishing authority to lawyers and teachers.

Rachel becomes more talkative and expresses her thoughts, feelings, and preferences as Tom shows interest in Rachel's construction of the problem and her views of self and other. This inspires Rachel to recount with real emotion how badly she feels about how others view her. She expresses her anger and hurt that her mother, sister, aunt, grandmother, and teachers think that she doesn't know what she's doing, in no uncertain terms.

Step 7. The next two steps are thinking steps. Based on the information gathered, therapists should consider how people prefer to be seen by others.

What is Rachel's preferred view? We infer from Rachel's comments about self and others that she prefers to see herself as tough, independent, able to manage her own affairs, smart enough to be in regular classes, and a champion of friends.

Step 8. Note the *gaps* between how people prefer to be seen and how they now see others seeing them. Problem-maintaining behavior emerges as people try to compensate for these disjunctive attributions.

At this point in the conversation with Rachel, it's clear that she now sees her mother, teachers, the school principal, other relatives, and even other therapists seeing her in ways that clash with her preferred view of self. Rachel grapples with this discrepancy by proving her toughness through fighting, by defying adult authority, by concealing her distress (and sadness) from adults, and by taking matters into her own hands.

Step 9. Discuss the evolution of the problem from the client's point of view. Inquire about the preproblem past. When did things go well? When did the client see others seeing him or her as he or she would like? At what point did things change? Was there a clear transition point or key event that triggered the onset of disjunctive views?

LUND: You're interested in getting back into regular classes? When were you last there?

RACHEL: When I was in elementary school, up until sixth grade.

LUND: How were things for you then?

RACHEL: Good.

LUND: What changed?

RACHEL: When I went to Roosevelt [Junior High School] . . . well . . . in sixth grade some girls thought they were tough, and they would pick on me and I wouldn't fight back. When I went to Roosevelt, I decided I wasn't letting no one pick on me and my friends.

LUND: I get the impression that you like to take charge of things for yourself.

RACHEL: Teachers let kids pick on each other, and they get mad at me when I help my friends, so I get mad at them.

LUND: What does your mom think of the teachers?

RACHEL: I don't know. She just listens to them, I don't like what they think of us.

LUND: What do they think of you?

RACHEL: They told my mom that where we live isn't a good place to raise a family. They said something about my sister and I having different fathers. Somehow they think that they are better.

LUND: It sounds like you don't want to hear much about that.

RACHEL: No, I don't.

New behavior emerges as Rachel tries to correct the discrepancy between how she wishes to be seen and how she thinks her classmates actually see her. We don't yet know how Rachel's mother responds to

The Evolving Problem

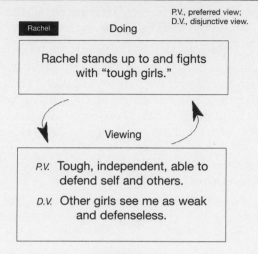

FIGURE 6.1.

the change in Rachel's behavior. It's clear, however, that school officials don't respond kindly to the new, no-nonsense Rachel.

In this conversational segment, Rachel pinpoints an important
time of transition in which she altered her approach to peers. In sixth
grade, Rachel felt that the other girls picked on her; she entered junior
high with a strong desire to prove her toughness. In Rachel's own
words, "I decided I wasn't letting no one pick on me and my friends."

Figure 6.1 links current behavior (doing) with key views of self
and other (viewing). In the viewing box, we highlight Rachel's preferred view of self and the views of others that contradict her preferences.[1] The arrows connecting viewing and doing show that it's the
experience of contradiction between how people prefer to be seen and
how they see others seeing them that propels problematic behavior.
The diagrams used in this book highlight only those preferences and
views related to the immediate problem. In this case, Rachel may have
a host of preferences that define how she would like to be seen as a
person, for example, smart, friendly, loyal, and competent. For Rachel,
however, there is something particularly meaningful about demon-
strating toughness in defending herself and her friends. It was this
preference that was challenged as Rachel entered junior high school.

As Rachel's teachers confronted Rachel about her behavior, she

[1]In this and subsequent figures, P. V. = preferred views, and D. V. = disjunctive views.

began talking back to them. As Rachel's misbehavior escalated, her mother appeared to Rachel to question her ability to manage her affairs. Rachel's upset was further fueled by her view that teachers "think they are better" than she and her mother. We can now diagram the actions and views that develop at this important time of transition, as Rachel entered junior high school (see Figure 6.2).

Although Tom has only spoken to Rachel for an hour, we have a clear assessment of the key views of self and other that contribute to problem development. We know about Rachel's preferences and intentions and how they were undermined at an important time of transition. As Rachel entered junior high school, she committed herself to disproving the theory that she was weak. She tried to assert herself as a tough kid who could stand up for her rights. Although she achieved this goal with her peers, disjunctive attributions mounted. Gradually, Rachel came to think that her teachers, her mother, her relatives, and professional helpers all perceived her as "incorrigible" and unable to manage her own affairs.

Understanding this flow of constructions, we're now poised to speak to Rachel's mother and compare her views of the evolving prob-

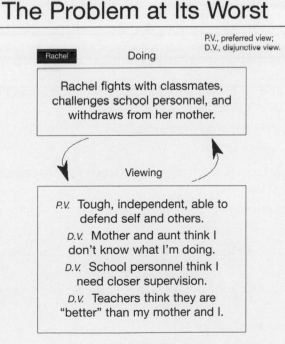

The Problem at Its Worst

P.V., preferred view;
D.V., disjunctive view.

Rachel   Doing

Rachel fights with classmates, challenges school personnel, and withdraws from her mother.

Viewing

P.V. Tough, independent, able to defend self and others.

D.V. Mother and aunt think I don't know what I'm doing.

D.V. School personnel think I need closer supervision.

D.V. Teachers think they are "better" than my mother and I.

FIGURE 6.2.

lem with Rachel's. Ultimately, our goal will be to help Rachel's mother converse differently with her daughter—to talk with her in a way that narrows the gap between how Rachel prefers to be seen and how she thinks others see her. To accomplish this goal, the therapist must begin talking with Rachel's mother in a way that suggests to her that he thinks that she's competent and capable. This process of aligning with preferences is enhanced by using information from the individual conversation with Rachel to suggest that Rachel values her mother's help and guidance.

Meeting with Rachel and her mother alone raises the issue of confidentiality. How do we decide what information to bring up in the session with Marion, and how do we get permission from Rachel to disclose that information? Typically, we explain our purpose as follows: "I'm interested in how your mother sees things. Would it be all right if I mentioned some of the things we talked about, so that I can get her view of the same events?" We then ask if there are specific things we shouldn't bring up in the conversation with Marion. We make it clear that our aim is not to tattle about unpleasant facts but to stick to perceptions, views and intentions.

We have a Columbo-like interest in "just the views," not a Sergeant Friday-like interest in "just the facts." Usually, people are more than happy to have us represent their "true" intentions, because they feel so badly misrepresented and misinterpreted. This was certainly the case with Rachel.

The conversation with Rachel's mother begins as follows:

LUND: I wound up having a longer talk with Rachel than I expected. I hope I didn't keep you waiting too long.

MARION: With her, it's easy to keep talking.

LUND: She's a talker?

MARION: No, I'm usually trying to convince her of something, and it takes awhile.

LUND: To get through?

MARION: Yes.

LUND: Actually she was doing a lot of the talking. She was quite talkative.

MARION: Well, that surprises me. Usually she'll clam up or get an attitude.

LUND: Has she always?

MARION: I'd say its been the last 2 years, with this more . . . "fighty attitude." She's made comments that if she doesn't like what people are saying, if other kids look her way, she's going to just pop them.

LUND: Does she?

MARION: A lot of times . . . yes . . . she was picked on a lot when she was younger and made up her mind that the kids are never going to pick on her again . . . and she doesn't care if she loses . . . she'll fight.

LUND: Just to make sure it doesn't go all one way.

MARION: Right.

The therapist is now hearing about the transition from the mother's point of view, when she first noticed Rachel standing up for herself and fighting her own battles. Marion and Rachel essentially agree with each other about when the problem began.

At this point the therapist digresses to connect more with Marion and understand her preferences, hopes, and intentions for herself and her daughter.

LUND: You've raised Rachel as a single parent?

MARION: Yes, I filed for divorce from her father and then found out that I was pregnant.

LUND: I don't know if you know this, but I don't have children, and I meet with a lot of single parents. I'm amazed that people do this on their own.

MARION: If you knew my ex-husband . . . things are easier this way.

LUND: He wouldn't have been helpful with the girls?

MARION: (*hesitating*) My ex-husband was an alcoholic, and I was a battered wife . . . and you wonder when the battered wife to the battered children would happen. I first believed the tears and promises, and finally got to the point of getting out. We went to a marriage counselor, who thought we were making great progress, but unless I lied to him and said things were getting better, I would be hit . . . it just wasn't good . . . I think I finally realized he was going to kill me.

LUND: So with a young daughter and a daughter on the way, you were able to get out?

MARION: Yes, I was pregnant and had a 5-year-old.

LUND: I guess Dad doesn't come around? He's out of the picture?

MARION: He's not in a position to be in the picture.

LUND: Oh, is he around here?

MARION: No, he's in another state.

LUND: Oh . . . he's . . .

MARION: To be perfectly honest, nobody outside the family knows this, but Rachel's father is in prison.

LUND: For something that happened after you split up?

MARION: Yeah, well . . . there has been more than one . . . this is the third time he is in prison. First he did 2 years and escaped, and had 1 year added. Then he was out for one month, then back for I don't know how long. Then the last time he was out for about 2 weeks and he was sentenced for 55 years.

LUND: Does Rachel know?

MARION: Yes, she found out. I told her, because, well, there was a time when he was getting out about 5 years ago. If he . . . I was afraid he was going to look me up.

LUND: That's a lot of worry.

MARION: I made do.

LUND: Sounds like you made do a lot!

MARION: I felt she had to know. As long as he is alive there is a danger to her.

LUND: A danger in the sense of . . . physical . . .

MARION: With the type of crime. The first was sexual assault . . . second was assault . . . last was sexual assault with attempted murder . . . he attempted to murder her so she could not identify him. Knowing him, she has to know his background and be able to take care of herself. There were a lot of threats . . . he said that he will come back and kill me when he can.

LUND: You've been interested in Rachel being able to stand up for herself, protect herself.

MARION: Yes, . . . I have.

It's no accident that Rachel's mother reveals information that she has told very few people over the years, information that sheds light on her positive intentions for her daughter. As Tom conveys his admiration that Rachel's mother reared Rachel as a single parent, Marion opens up about the status of Rachel's father. We learn later that Marion is accustomed to being criticized and has felt ashamed about her selection of a husband and father and what became of him. It's helpful to have this information about the broad narrative picture, because we can now see *why* Marion may have preferred to raise a daughter who could fight her own battles. Perhaps she thought Rachel would need toughness to stand up to her father if he were ever to return to the scene.

We now want to talk with Marion about how she regarded Rachel's intentions when Rachel moved on to junior high school. This is a good time to use information obtained from our conversation with Rachel to reframe her positive intentions at this important time of transition.

LUND: You seem to have raised a youngster who is very interested in asserting herself, taking charge, not being victimized. She talked about taking a stand about this somewhere around fifth, sixth, or seventh grade. Do you recall?

MARION: Actually I do. I remember she was being picked on by one girl in fifth grade, an older and much bigger girl at the bus stop. One day I could tell something was going to happen, I don't know why . . . but I followed her . . . actually, I brought a camera . . . this girl started pushing, and Rachel knocked her down and hit her a few times. I caught it on camera, for proof, just in case someone said Rachel started it.

LUND: What did Rachel think of your taking a picture?

MARION: I think she was pleased that I supported her.

LUND: Are you able to support her now?

MARION: I don't know. I guess that's a good question.

LUND: Why?

MARION: I would like to support her. I would like to do something, but she doesn't seem to listen. She's not interested in hearing from me.

LUND: Was she ever?

MARION: A long while ago.

LUND: You were close?

MARION: We used to be close. We did things together. (*smiling warmly*) In fact, she was my shadow. I used to turn around and she'd be doing just what I was doing.

LUND: When did this change?

MARION: Actually, it probably was around fifth or sixth grade, or maybe junior high school, when things really began getting worse. She seemed to get a real fighty attitude. She wouldn't listen to anyone.

Isn't it interesting that in the early stages of problem development Rachel's mother seemed pleased with Rachel's "fighty attitude"? She even went so far as to photograph her daughter when she was engaged in battle to document the occasion. Marion has now filled in a good deal of the story about a daughter who approached adolescence with a keen interest in "standing up for herself," and about a parent who felt her daughter needed toughness to protect herself, possibly even from her own father. We can now see that Rachel's intentions were to follow in her mother's footsteps, to be her "shadow," as Marion so poetically put it. How painful it must be for Rachel to think that her mother is now deferring to others, and for her mother to think that Rachel doesn't need her guidance anymore.

With the information we now have from Rachel's mother, we know enough to complete the doing–viewing cycle started before, filling in Marion's half of the diagram (see Figure 6.3). As you can see from this diagram, in the early stages of problem evolution Rachel's "fighty" approach was encouraged by her mother. Rachel saw her mother seeing her as tough, strong, and competent, which spurred Rachel on to do more of the same. Somewhere along the way, however, this all went awry as Rachel's combative behavior escalated and

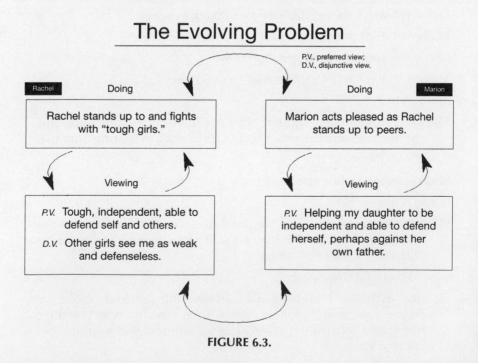

The Evolving Problem

P.V., preferred view;
D.V., disjunctive view.

Rachel — Doing

Rachel stands up to and fights with "tough girls."

Viewing

P.V. Tough, independent, able to defend self and others.

D.V. Other girls see me as weak and defenseless.

Marion — Doing

Marion acts pleased as Rachel stands up to peers.

Viewing

P.V. Helping my daughter to be independent and able to defend herself, perhaps against her own father.

FIGURE 6.3.

Marion felt helpless to contain her. As school officials reacted sternly to Rachel and Marion, Marion reversed her approach.

She began to reconnote Rachel's behavior as unproductive and challenge her about her ability to manage her own affairs. With this, Rachel upped the aggressive behavior yet another notch, which led to more severe punishment by school officials and more criticism of the family. Marion grew more uncertain about what to do, resorting to desperate measures such as the "endless-restriction" approach and deferring to relatives and other outside resources. Once Rachel saw her mother as kowtowing to outsiders, things really intensified. Seeing her once strong mother—who stood up to and left her abusive father—now turn weak and deferential must have felt to Rachel like the very foundation of the family was about to crumble.

The doing–viewing cycle at its worst can now be drawn (see Figure 6.4).

At its worst, Rachel thinks that nearly everyone views her in ways

The Problem at Its Worst

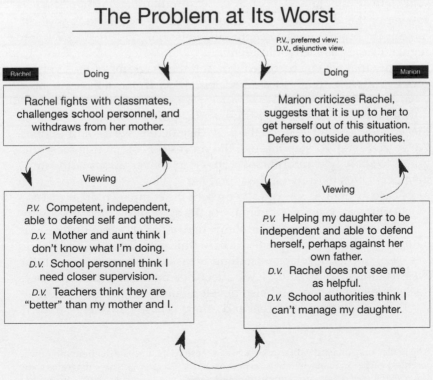

FIGURE 6.4.

that clash with her preferred view. The experience of this gap fuels more of the same take-charge, stand-up-for-yourself, defiant behavior, which in turn shapes how Marion approaches talking with Rachel. Mom, too, thinks that nearly everyone views her in ways that run counter to her preferences. As Marion sees her daughter, school officials, relatives, and counselors regarding her as a bad mother who can't manage her daughter, her confidence wanes. Thus, she defers to others, while conveying anger and disappointment in Rachel for not managing herself adequately. When Tom first meets with Rachel and Marion, no one is managing very well, and we have a family on the verge of not being a family anymore.

Simply look at the doing–viewing cycle, and the goal becomes clear. We would like to see Rachel's mother reclaim her position as guide and confidant to Rachel. We'd like to see her take charge of her daughter's behavior in a calm, matter-of-fact way; not to defer so much to others; and, to appeal to Rachel to take charge of her affairs so that other authority figures back off and hand the controls back to the family. We assume that if Mom alters her approach to Rachel, Rachel will, in turn, alter how she perceives her mother viewing her. The narrowing of this disjunctive gap should influence Rachel to behave differently, to tone down her aggressive behavior, and to get back into regular classes, as she would prefer.

Now that we've proceeded through the diagrams of the evolving problem cycle through to the problem at its worst, let's summarize what we have portrayed. We've attempted to show diagrammatically how a problem evolves, intensifies, and rigidifies over time, based on the emergence and continuation of disjunctive views and actions. We've gone step by step through the process of completing these diagrams to show how information derived in conversations with family members helps in drawing these problem cycles. As we proceed with more case examples, we typically present the completed diagrams as a whole unit—as a succinct summary of the story of problem evolution.

The completed diagrams show that circular, more-of-the-same patterns of thought *and* action occur within and between people.[2] In this case, Rachel develops unsettling ideas about herself through the eyes of others, and these views affect her behavior. Marion notices Rachel's new behavior and also develops unsettling ideas about herself through the eyes of Rachel and others. These new views, in turn,

---

[2]The reader may notice the difference between these problem-cycle diagrams and those described earlier in reviewing the MRI approach (see Chapter 2). These diagrams show how viewing *and* doing intertwine as problems evolve and revolve. The MRI diagrams depict behavioral problem cycles only.

affect changes in Marion's behavior. Rachel notices her mother's new behavior and intensifies her defiant behavior. As this problem cycle churns with more and more momentum, views and actions narrow and become more rigid. People notice only the actions of others that support disjunctive attributions.[3]

In the completed diagrams, arrows are used to connect meaning and action (or viewing and doing) at the level of self and at the level of interaction. At times of transition, people begin to act differently. This news of difference is interpreted by others in ways that contradict preferred views, setting in motion more-of-the-same patterns of viewing and doing.

KEEPING IN MIND ALL OF THESE VIEWS

In addition to mapping the doing and viewing elements of a problem cycle, we've also found it useful to organize the key views of self and other into a table, which we call the "matrix of views." This matrix permits disjunctive views (linked to the creation of the problem) to stand out in bold relief. As we listen to the stories people tell about their lives that inform their current predicament, there are numerous views that come out, and these views can be difficult to keep track of. Not only is the matrix a good tracking device, but also it can be helpful when our conversations with people bog down or evoke unexpected resistance. These are good times to consult the matrix, to check out whether we have missed a key view that might help us go after new information or adjust our approach.

Filling out the matrix is an exercise in charting the narrative landscape. People tell us lots of stories about key people in their lives. They often bounce around in time, offering vignettes from the distant and recent past, as well as the problem-saturated present. Some of these stories are relevant to problem development, and some aren't. Those stories that clarify how people wish to be seen by each other—that highlight the emergence of disjunctive attributions—are the ones we want to pursue in the conversation. From each person's individual, narrative account, we try to cull out the key views of self and other that shape the current predicament, and enter these views into the matrix.

---

[3]In this sense, we could also say that views and actions are contained within a problem-sustaining frame. These problematic frames are supported by certain stories and disconfirmed by others. The concepts of frame and story are difficult to portray pictorially: however, in the next section, we show how another tool for assessment (the matrix of views) depicts the concept of frames.

Let's take a look at a blank matrix (see Figure 6.5). You'll see that on the top of the grid we list the members of the family caught in the web of the problem. Goolishian and Anderson (1987) referred to this unit of people as the "problem-determined system." In this sense, the "family" that we see in therapy and collect views from are those people in current interaction around the problem whose actions and views affect the course of the problem. Thus, the problem determines the system more so than the system determines the problem. In this case, our "system" consists of two people—Rachel and her mother. These two people talk about numerous others who have influenced the course of the problem. However, we believe that if Rachel and her mother change their approach to conversing with each other and to important others inside and outside the family, the problem can be resolved without involving other people directly in the therapeutic conversation.

This blank matrix appears as a table with a border around it and a series of boxes within it. This pictorial image evokes the concept of frame. Family members organize their own experience by creating borders or boundaries around events and situations. An event such as Rachel's fighting in school might be framed at one point in time as an indication that she is standing up for herself and asserting her own independence. When her mother sees the behavior within this frame, she also sees herself as a competent mother who has helped her daughter "toughen up," and sees her daughter seeing her as a good mother who

Vantage points	Family members			
Preferred view of self				
View of significant others				
View of family of origin				
View of therapist or other helpers				

FIGURE 6.5. Matrix of views.

has helped her get to this point. At the time Rachel's mother took a picture of Rachel fighting with another girl, she was looking at Rachel's behavior within this preferred, nonproblematic frame.

The key views that appear in the matrix, however, reflect how people see each other *now*, within the narrow problem-saturated framework of current interaction. What will get recorded in the boxes of the matrix are current views, such as "Mom views Rachel as not managing her own affairs very well," or "Mom views Rachel viewing her as a bad mother who has failed to provide proper guidance." The boxes that appear in the matrix are like the tiny little boxes that people see their worlds within when they feel stuck and boxed in. These are the key views that we hope to change in the therapeutic conversation, and we'll change them by shifting people's attention away from these "boxed in" views and toward stories and experiences that confirm their preferences and positive intentions.

The first box in the matrix represents each person's *preferred view of self* (see Figure 6.6). We glean from each person's individual narrative account of the problem how that person would like to be seen by the important others in his or her sphere. We can then compare the preferred attributions recorded in this box with notations in the other boxes of the matrix. The other boxes of the matrix pertain more to how people now see important others in their immediate and historical field, and how they see those others seeing them.

The second box in the matrix is labeled "View of Significant Others" (see Figure 6.7). Here we take note of how family members view the others in their immediate sphere. Also included in this box of the matrix are views about living others who may not be in current interaction around the problem, but play an important role in the broader narrative picture. For example, in this case, we might take note of Mother's view of Rachel's biological father. Although he is now in prison and not directly affecting the current family interaction, the narrative theme around toughness, resiliency, and standing up for oneself against others was shaped by the father's participation in, and removal from, the family.

Rachel	Marion
Tough, independent, able to defend self and others.	Helping daughter be independent and able to defend herself, perhaps against her own father.

FIGURE 6.6. Preferred view of self.

Rachel	Marion
D. V.—School personnel think I need closer supervision. **D. V.**—Teachers think they are better than my mother and I.	**D. V.**—Rachel does not see me as helpful. **D. V.**—School authorities think I can't manage my daughter. *Rachel's father is a danger to Rachel.

FIGURE 6.7. View of significant others.

We might note, for example, that Mom now views Rachel as needing to defend herself, perhaps against her own father. Since this idea might contribute to Marion's encouraging her daughter's toughness and confidence in defending herself, it looms as a key construction. In this way, the matrix can be used as a navigational guide for the therapeutic conversation, alerting the therapist to reframing and restorying possibilities. (Note that we place an asterisk next to this view of the father, to signify its strong emotional loading and to cue us to use this view at some point in the therapeutic conversation.)

In the third box of the matrix, we shift the narrative vantage point to consider family of origin (see Figure 6.8). In cases involving children and parents, we're particularly interested in how parents see their own parents being parents. Do they wish to follow in their parents' footsteps? Do they have a strong preference to parent differently? Also, how do they see their own parents seeing them: as ineffective or competent, loyal or disloyal? We consider the children's view of their parents and, if relevant, how they see their grandparents seeing their parents, and how they see their grandparents seeing them.

In this case, Rachel views her mother and her aunt seeing her as unable to manage her affairs. We do not have information about Marion's view of her parents or their view of her.

In the last box of the matrix, we take note of how people view therapists and other professional helpers (see Figure 6.9). In this case, Rachel was angry at previous helpers. She saw them as aligning with

Rachel	Marion
D. V.—My aunt thinks I don't know what I'm doing.	

FIGURE 6.8. View of family of origin.

Rachel	Marion
Previous therapist thought I didn't know what I was doing.	Helpers cannot help unless Rachel wants them to.

FIGURE 6.9. View of therapist or other helpers.

her teachers, her mother, and other adults, in regarding her as unable to manage her independence. Knowing about this view helped the therapist reframe Rachel's antitherapy stance as a sign that she was her "own person" and knew what she was doing. By assuming this position, the therapist connected with Rachel's preferences. Soon, Rachel began talking openly with him, despite her misgivings about being in therapy.

At this point, we have the entire matrix of views (see Figure 6.10). We can now use this table as a navigational guide in managing a helpful conversation. In the next chapter, we'll show how the key views that appear in these boxes can be altered by restorying the evolution of the problem and by reframing current behavior.

Vantage points	Rachel	Marion
Preferred view of self	Tough, independent, able to defend self and others	Helping my daughter be independent and able to defend herself, perhaps against her own father.
View of significant others	**D. V.**—School personnel think I need closer supervision. **D. V.**—Teachers think they are better than my mother and I.	**D. V.**—Rachel does not see me as helpful. **D. V.**—School authorities think I can't manage my daughter. *Rachel's father is a danger to Rachel.
View of family of origin	My aunt thinks I don't know what I'm doing.	
View of therapist or other helpers	Previous therapist thought I didn't know what I was doing.	Helpers cannot help unless Rachel wants them to.

FIGURE 6.10. Complete matrix of views.

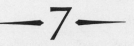

The Strategy of Conversation, Part III: Steps to Narrative Solutions

et's examine the steps the therapist takes to develop an alternative explanation for the evolving problem that brings about a solution. Although these steps coincide with the "assessment" steps outlined earlier, we now emphasize the elements of therapeutic conversation that inspire behavior change.

Step 1. The therapist locates stories that are in line with each person's preferred view and contradict the narrow range of disjunctive views and actions that maintain the problem.

Step 2. The therapist encourages the circulation of these preferred stories with other family members.

We left our story of 14-year-old Rachel and her mother Marion with clear ideas about how Rachel turned "incorrigible" in the eyes of adults. The problem evolved as Rachel entered junior high school and began fighting with classmates. It was then that her teachers and mother changed how they regarded and treated her. Rachel described how her mother, who once trusted and consoled her, now deferred to relatives and strangers about her private business. Rachel had come to see her mother as having little respect for her, which led to further defiance and withdrawal.

THE PREPROBLEM PAST

The therapist shifts the conversation away from this present, stuck interaction to the preproblem past. He creates a climate of nostalgia, reviving memories of times when Rachel and her mother viewed each other in preferred ways.

LUND: Do you and Mom do much together?

RACHEL: Not really. We're always mad.

LUND: Did you ever?

RACHEL: A while ago.

LUND: What?

RACHEL: My mom goes for walks. I used to go.

LUND: Anything else?

RACHEL: Shopping.

LUND: How was that for you?

RACHEL: It was okay. I don't want to talk to her anymore.

LUND: It sounds like you used to like to talk to her, but now she tells everybody your business.

RACHEL: That's right.

LUND: Was she interested in what you had to say?

RACHEL: I guess so. It seemed like it.

LUND: Were you interested in what she had to say?

RACHEL: Yeah, why?

LUND: I had the impression that your mom liked it better when you used to talk, . . . you liked it better when you used to talk, . . . but you and Mom aren't talking.

RACHEL: I guess that's true.

Having obtained this alternative story of the mother–daughter relationship, the therapist now circulates that story in conversation with the mother. The therapist brings Marion back to a time when Rachel listened to her and respected her guidance.

LUND: You mentioned that you thought Rachel wasn't interested in your ideas. I think you said that Rachel wasn't "interested in hearing from you."

MARION: No, she isn't interested in hearing from me anymore.

LUND: She was at one time?

MARION: Actually, when she was much younger I used to call her my shadow . . . it was a bit much, actually . . . I would be trying to get something done. I'd turn around and she'd be right behind me. I'd almost trip over her.

LUND: What was she doing?

MARION: She was imitating me.

LUND: Rachel mentioned that she liked to walk with you.

MARION: For years we took walks after dinner. She used to run out of the house after me.

LUND: She used to look up to you.

MARION: She did . . .

ALTERNATIVE EXPLANATIONS

Step 3. Therapist and client develop an alternative explanation for the evolution of the problem, which permits current problem-maintaining behavior to be reframed. This alternative explanation fits with how people prefer to be seen by others and inspires new action.

Step 4. Family members begin to view important others regarding them in ways that fit their preferences. The narrowing of this gap, or disjunction, promotes less of the same problem-maintaining behavior.

The conversation with Rachel's mother continues.

LUND: I had the impression that Rachel liked that. . . . It's curious that somewhere along the line it began looking like she wasn't interested any longer.

MARION: I guess she wanted to be her own person.

LUND: That makes sense. At some point I guess she decided to be even more like you—independent, taking charge, standing up for people, like you do for your children.

MARION: I don't know what you mean.

LUND: Well, she seems to view her "fighty attitude" as being independent, taking care of her own business. Unless I'm mistaken, a lot of her conflict comes when she stands up for herself, and also when she stands up for or, from her point of view, protects friends.

MARION: That's an interesting way to look at it.

LUND: What do you think?

MARION: I may have encouraged some of that.

LUND: She seems to have listened.

MARION: It doesn't seem like that when I try to talk to her.

LUND: I mentioned to Rachel that I had the impression that you both liked it better when you used to talk, when she was interested in talking to you, interested in your input . . . but you don't talk now.

MARION: You think that she's still interested in hearing what I have to say?

LUND: Yes.

MARION: I'm getting the impression that I did too good a job of making her independent and teaching her to stand up for herself.

As Rachel's mother recalls stories from the preproblem past (when Rachel had "acted like her shadow" and tried to imitate her), she and the therapist begin to weave an alternative explanation for Rachel's recent defiant behavior. Mom entertains the new (and less disjunctive) idea that Rachel's stubborn resistance to adult guidance is simply an outgrowth of her desire to be strong like her mother. She begins to see that as Rachel approached adolescence, she got carried away with trying to be tough and resilient. Perhaps Rachel envisioned a future in which she, too, would have to fight battles to maintain her dignity.

This alternative explanation confirms Marion's preference to be a caring mother whom her daughter looks to for direction. With this, Marion begins to consider a different approach to her daughter's troublesome behavior. She thinks about resuming her role as guide and protector, helping Rachel to pick and choose the right battles, and to channel her independent spirit so that she may become the competent adult she wants to become.

The conversation between the therapist and Rachel's mother continues with a focus on how to guide Rachel. We are now moving into the realm of doing, of pattern-breaking action.

LUND: How do you choose the right battles? For instance, Rachel seemed angry at the teachers who were saying you're raising her in a bad environment.

MARION: Oh, you know how people say things. Teachers have their own problems. I can't take those things too seriously. If you react, you only make things worse. I stand up when it's more important.

LUND: I wonder if Rachel knew that you didn't really care much for what the teacher said, that you stand up in your own quiet way, and that by not reacting you avoided making things worse.

MARION: She needs to choose her battles.

Step 5. Once disjunctive gaps in perception narrow, family members begin to engage in helpful conversations with each other. These new conversations reinforce emerging solutions.

GENERATIVE CONVERSATIONS

Equipped with a preferred explanation for the problem, Marion went home and talked with Rachel about one of their recent meetings with the teachers that preceded Rachel's suspension from school. Mom started out respectfully by asking Rachel what she thought about the teacher's comments. As Rachel offered her opinion that she would have liked to hit the teacher, Marion listened quietly. She then acknowledged that it was upsetting that a teacher would speak condescendingly to a student and parent, but emphasized how she wasn't personally offended by the inappropriate comments. Marion explained that ignoring people can be the best way to stand up for yourself in some situations. When Rachel countered that she would have liked to punch the teacher in the face, Mom calmly stuck to her position, citing other incidents in which she had maintained her own pride by refusing to "stoop to the other person's level." The conversation continued with Rachel asking about other times in her mother's life when she felt she had to "stand up" for herself.

Tom then spoke with Rachel about this recent (helpful) conversation at home.

LUND: Your mom mentioned that she spoke with you about the meeting with that teacher that made you angry.

RACHEL: I would have punched her if I was my mom.

LUND: What did Mom think of that idea?

RACHEL: She actually agreed for once that the lady shouldn't be able to say those things, that I had a right to be mad.

LUND: She agreed that you should stand up to people when they do those things.

RACHEL: Yeah, I guess . . . I guess she did.

LUND: So how come she didn't punch her?

RACHEL: Because she said then the teacher would look good . . . she would be in trouble.

Step 6. As things change, views of self and other, and actions, become more flexible and less restricted. People lose sight of the idea that a problem really exists, and they no longer locate its blame or cause in deficiencies of self or other.

Tom also spoke with Marion about the effects of empowering conversations; clarifying what worked and why.

LUND: Rachel seemed pleased that you "agreed with her," that you thought you should stand up to people who say things like the teacher. She seems to want to talk more when she feels you see her making sense.

MARION: I didn't realize that what I said mattered very much. I was asking Rachel what she would like to come from this court appearance.

LUND: Had you ever asked her about that before?

MARION: I don't think so . . . I think I warned her, and I told her I was upset. I don't think I asked what *she* wanted.

LUND: What did she say?

MARION: She said that she wanted court to be over so that she could go back to her regular classes.

LUND: What did you say?

MARION: I said that I wanted her to remain at home and would love to see her in regular classes.

LUND: Had you and she ever spoken about that before?

MARION: I'm not sure—we mostly argued about what she was doing.

LUND: It's interesting, you seem to be talking with her about what she would like, and it doesn't sound very different from what you would like.

MARION: I don't think we've talked much about what we would like with each other.

LUND: I asked Rachel why a bright, competent young lady who wanted to take care of her own business, and to be in regular class, was not realizing that goal.

MARION: What did she say?

LUND: She didn't really answer it, but I think she was thinking about it.

Interestingly, Mother began to take over where the therapist left off by asking her daughter lots of preference questions, and joining with her as a competent person who truly wanted to be independent. Therapists model how to conduct helpful conversations by expressing interest in people's preferences and positive intentions. Rachel now had the experience of two adults (therapist and mother) thinking of her and conversing with her in ways she preferred. Had the therapist spoken with Marion in a confrontational manner about what she was doing wrong, Marion, in turn, might have spoken with Rachel in a confrontational manner about what she was doing wrong. Helpful and unhelpful conversations have a contagious effect.

After the Family Court judge ruled that Rachel should be placed on probation and returned to the same special class as before, Marion talked more with Rachel about how to handle her teachers and probation officer. Mother reclaimed her role as guide and confidant. She even started to pose the "mystery question" to Rachel. Instead of getting angry and accusing Rachel of being obnoxious, she'd simply ask Rachel why someone who wanted to get back to regular classes would talk back to teachers. Or, she'd gently challenge Rachel by asking her why she let the teachers get the best of her. Although she dispensed with the rumpled raincoat, Rachel's mother began to play Columbo with her own daughter.

Beyond being curious, nonjudgmental, and respectful to her daughter, Rachel's mother also backed this up with appropriate discipline. Instead of resorting to desperate measures such as "endless grounding," Marion would insist that Rachel help her with work around the house, which had the side benefit of reinforcing further cooperation and cohesion in the mother–daughter relationship. Rachel didn't put up too much of a fuss about these consequences, because it became clear that her mother hadn't given up on her and regarded her as capable and competent. Thus, the sequence of generative conversations went as follows:

1. The therapist talked to the daughter and the mother in a way that aligned with their preferences, hopes, and positive intentions.

2. The therapist circulated the daughter's preferences to the mother as he and Rachel's mother began to weave an alternative explanation for the evolution of the problem.
3. The mother began to talk with her daughter in a more helpful way by connecting with her preferences, hopes, and positive intentions. She indicated that she would love to see Rachel in regular classes, and as not needing to be under the watchful eye of the court or probation. She also began to help Rachel reach her goals by guiding her about how to act toward teachers and other authority figures, and by applying matter-of-fact consequences for misbehavior.
4. As Rachel began to see the therapist and her mother seeing her in preferred ways, she began to alter her own conversational approach with peers, teachers, school officials, and other adults.

The therapist followed up by talking with Rachel about the recent changes that had taken place. This was done to solidify the connection between "new meaning and new action."

LUND: Mom seems to be getting tough.

RACHEL: What do you mean?

LUND: Well, she told me that she's making you work around the house.

RACHEL: It's not very hard.

LUND: No?

RACHEL: No, but I'm mad that she *makes me* do it.

LUND: I'll bet you are! Why do you do it?

RACHEL: Because I have to. Mom makes me.

LUND: I wonder why she got into this rather than the endless grounding?

RACHEL: I don't know. It makes more sense.

LUND: More sense?

RACHEL: Yes, if I do something wrong, if I overreact to things, Mom gets mad. She says she wants me to get back to regular classes, and she is going to make it tough on me if I don't.

LUND: I don't get it. I thought you wanted to get out of special classes.

RACHEL: I do.

LUND: So what does punishment have to do with that?

RACHEL: Mom thinks I can get out of the special classes, so she punishes me for doing things she thinks will keep me in them.

LUND: That's interesting ... that makes sense. If you don't manage your business in a way that gets you what you want, Mom will help motivate you.

RACHEL: I wouldn't look at it like that.

In the past, Rachel would have expressed disdain for any new approach to "punishment." Now she comes close to defending her mother's "get tough" methods, although she stops short of admitting they're helpful. The reason Marion's new behavior is "reframed" by Rachel is that she now sees her mother as on her side and striving for the same goals. Rachel sees Marion as providing guidance and reinforcing her strengths, not as meting out harsh punishments and emphasizing her flaws.

Therapy concluded as Rachel's mother took over from the therapist as manager of the conversation. As Marion lent power to Rachel through confidence building and gentle direction, Rachel's behavior changed. As Rachel began talking openly with her mother, Marion noticed that Rachel valued her.

After 10 sessions (over a 6-month period of counseling), Rachel had stopped getting into fights with other girls at school and refrained from battling with her teachers. When her grades and behavior improved, she was allowed to return to regular classes, just as she and her mother hoped. Rachel's probation officer backed off from monitoring Rachel and Marion closely and simply asked for another progress report in a year's time. Rachel's mother took over the reins of conversation with her daughter, as other adults, including the therapist, took a backseat.

In the early stages of therapy, Tom met with Rachel and Marion individually. As things improved and conversational patterns changed, Tom met with mother and daughter together to affirm what they had accomplished and to consolidate their vision of the future. The final session was held with Rachel and Marion together, as the therapist (symbolically) passed the baton over to the mother.

We can now diagram the basic elements of a *narrative solution* (see Figure 7.1). You can see how solutions emerge when family members begin to think and act in ways that suit them. They reconstruct the actions and intentions of self and other in ways that confirm preferred views.[1] As the gap narrows between how people wish to perceive

---

[1]In the viewing box, the designation P.V. = preferred views, and N.D.V. = nondisjunctive views. The arrows connecting the viewing to doing boxes show how new meaning becomes linked to new action.

A Narrative Solution

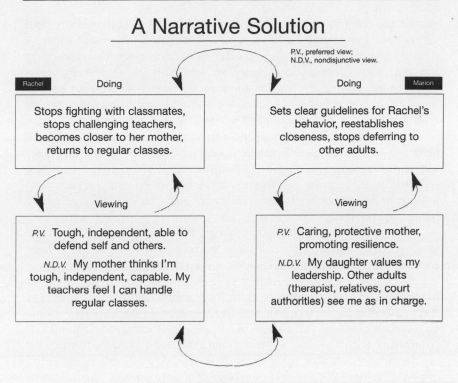

P.V., preferred view;
N.D.V., nondisjunctive view.

Rachel | Doing

Stops fighting with classmates, stops challenging teachers, becomes closer to her mother, returns to regular classes.

Doing | Marion

Sets clear guidelines for Rachel's behavior, reestablishes closeness, stops deferring to other adults.

Viewing

P.V. Tough, independent, able to defend self and others.

N.D.V. My mother thinks I'm tough, independent, capable. My teachers feel I can handle regular classes.

Viewing

P.V. Caring, protective mother, promoting resilience.

N.D.V. My daughter values my leadership. Other adults (therapist, relatives, court authorities) see me as in charge.

FIGURE 7.1.

themselves and how they think others regard them (viewing), people change problem-maintaining patterns of behavior (doing).

THE CASE OF THE MISSING VIEW

In this three-chapter series on the strategy of conversation, we've outlined steps to be taken, positions to be assumed, and information to be gathered in managing conversations that help people get beyond their problems. We've also offered tools for careful assessment (the matrix of views and the doing–viewing cycles) to demonstrate that there can be a method in navigating a helpful conversation. Restorying and reframing aren't magic. Rather, these conversational "interventions" develop out of information we glean from the stories people tell us about their lives, and the information becomes gleanable only when therapists assume a particular position with people—one that enjoins their preferences and good intentions.

When we talk about the art of therapeutic conversation in this systematic fashion, we also feel compelled to tell the other side of the story. Because change happens through a process no more magical than an ordinary conversation, there is plenty of room for error. What happens when things don't work so smoothly, when the therapist misses a step, or forgets to elicit a key view? Can these tools for assessment also come in handy after we accidentally step on a land mine (or a preferred view) and evoke massive resistance from people?

Let's consider a case that didn't proceed like clockwork, to show how trying to understand people's views can be a slippery business. Yet, if you maintain a respectful position with your clients and stay with the task of unraveling the mystery of problem constructions and getting at key views that surround problems, you can often rebound from your mistakes.

The case of 9-year-old Adam Freer and his parents shows how attending to the wide array of views in the matrix of views helps to steer a wayward therapeutic conversation back on track.

Tom was asked to evaluate young Adam, who was diagnosed as having epilepsy and attention-deficit/hyperactivity disorder and was on medication for both conditions. In an ongoing struggle to help their son, Adam's parents took him to numerous doctors and therapists. Adam met with the family's physician on a regular basis to monitor his medication after he went through extensive evaluations by teams of pediatric neurologists and psychologists at two major medical centers. Mr. and Mrs. Freer also worked closely with the special education department at their son's school. They wanted to consult a therapist about behavioral problems that lingered despite the medication, which had helped Adam's epilepsy and allowed him to focus better on his schoolwork. Adam became extremely agitated when asked to take on responsibilities that seemed well within his capabilities. The Freers requested that Tom see Adam a few times to help figure out what was getting in the way of his completion of these tasks, and to help them come up with some better ways to approach the problem.

After meeting with Adam and his parents in various combinations on three occasions, it seemed clear that lack of confidence loomed as a reasonable explanation for Adam's reluctance to take on responsibilities of which he was capable. Adam preferred to see himself as a regular kid who was just as competent as the others in his class. Yet, he viewed his teachers, his parents, and his brother (who did well in school) as all perceiving him as inept. He felt badly about being different. One event that had a significant impact on Adam was an innocent lecture given by his third grade teacher about the nature of independence and responsibility. She warned the children in her class about the weighty responsibilities that lay ahead in fourth grade, and lectured them that third grade was the time to become more independent. This talk struck a responsive chord with Adam, who came home filled with enthusiasm about doing things for himself. Mr. and Mrs. Freer were pleased and allowed Adam more freedom to manage responsibilities on his own.

As Adam's well-meaning parents began to give him more rope in an effort to build his confidence, he began to tie himself into knots, leaving his parents weary, exasperated, and at the end of *their* ropes. Mr. and Mrs. Freer were used to watching Adam closely, sitting down with him as he did his homework, staying in the room with him as he got dressed for school, reminding him often to brush his teeth and comb his hair, sometimes even doing these things for him. They were encouraged recently by the medical experts that it was okay to back off a little. Since Adam was on medication to control his seizures and hyperactivity, the doctors felt he could now handle many of these everyday responsibilities on his own. Unfortunately, as Adam's parents backed off, Adam began neglecting his personal hygiene and forgetting to do his homework. When Mr. and Mrs. Freer questioned him about these oversights, Adam told them not to worry, that it was done or would get done, and to just leave him alone. Later his parents would find out that nothing was accomplished. Feeling deliberately misled, the parents would reprimand Adam for being irresponsible, untrustworthy, and manipulative. Such scoldings made Adam fly into a rage, slamming doors and screaming at the top of his lungs, winding up finally sobbing in his parents' arms. He'd shake like a leaf as his parents apologized for upsetting him and tried their best to comfort him.

A FAST AND LOOSE REFRAME

Having put together this story of the evolving problem, Tom felt he was ready to intervene. It seemed that Mr. and Mrs. Freer were competent, caring parents who were trying to do the best for their child, a child with limitations that were hard to accept and difficult to manage. Tom figured that he'd align with the parents as capable, then steer them toward a solution that involved more vigilance, guidance, and confidence building.

Tom jumped in by informing the Freers of their son's positive intentions, saying that he was a good boy who wanted to do well but seemed to have a confidence problem. Tom was about to connect with the parents' preferred view, but before he could utter another word, Mrs. Freer started to cry. The tears turned to anger as she laced into

Tom for his insensitivity. "You don't understand how hard we've tried to build Adam's confidence." Tom sat speechless, trying to absorb this sudden intense reaction. Before he could say anything, Mrs. Freer glared at him and stormed out of the office with her husband close behind, looking slightly embarrassed by his wife's outburst but trying his best to stand by her. Her parting words were hard to forget. "If I want to be criticized, I can get plenty of that for free. I don't have to pay for it," she said.

For several days Tom kept thinking: Criticized? How was I sounding critical? Didn't I connect with Mrs. Freer's preferences? Hadn't I set the stage for the therapeutic conversation? How could these parents possibly see me as blaming them? After all, I'm a postmodern therapist who maintains a nonhierarchical, nonblaming, nonimpositional, and collaborative therapeutic stance. Didn't they know that?

GETTING THE WHOLE STORY

It was time for a consultation. We took some time to step back from the situation to see what Tom had missed, and in the process developed further this idea about a "matrix of views." We decided that if Tom got another chance to speak to the family, he could begin by reclaiming his own good intentions and by inviting the parents to help him figure out what he missed. Then, maybe the mystery of Mrs. Freer's sudden and unexplainable outburst might just as suddenly become explainable.

Remarkably, Mr. and Mrs. Freer did call for another appointment. Tom began the next session by telling them how badly he felt that he appeared critical of them. He clarified that he actually thought that they had done a wonderful job with Adam, getting the best possible help for their son. "What was it I said that made you feel criticized?" he asked.

With this, the parents informed Tom about what he missed in his rather cursory gathering of views. (They might as well have said, "See boxes two and three in the matrix of views! You forgot to get the views of other family members!") They described their feeling that all four grandparents and other relatives saw Adam as a good little boy who meant well. They felt criticized by them for not giving him enough love and reassurance. Apparently the grandparents saw the parents as being much too hard on Adam. When Tom launched into his "Adam has good intentions and wants to do well" dissertation, the parents heard him saying, "You're not giving him enough love and reassurance." Thus, they saw the therapist *not* as connecting with them as competent parents, but rather as joining with the grandparents and other family members in seeing them as uncaring and insensitive. The intensity of the parents' reaction spoke to the intensity of emotion behind their experience of disjunction—to just how badly they felt about being criticized by members of their own family as they tried their best to help manage their 9-year-old son.

Though Tom's intention was to align with the parents' preferences, obviously he had failed. If anything, they felt more "aligned against" than "aligned with," and the conversation was going nowhere. Once Tom clarified that he saw Adam as a challenging child to help and to protect, and that he saw the parents as managing rather well under trying circumstances, the conversation was able to move along with greater ease. In fact, as the parents began to see the therapist seeing them in line with their preferences, Mrs. Freer opened up about an important story that she had rarely talked about with people. She felt that Adam's epilepsy had been triggered by an unfortunate accident that happened when he was an infant. Her view of the accident was that it occurred because she hadn't watched him closely enough, which left her forever feeling like a neglectful parent.

Ultimately, Tom was able to incorporate the grandparents' view of the problem into a more helpful reconstruction of problem evolution. The alternative story that emerged was that Adam was thrown off track by the third grade teacher's lecture on responsibility, and that this idea that his parents should let up on structure and guidance left him frightened and shaky. The implication of this new construction was that the grandparents' theory about how to manage Adam was ill-advised. For a young boy who had epileptic seizures and attention problems, who had benefited by his parents' vigilance and insistence on proper medical care, to be suddenly given a "You're-on-you-own, you-can-do-it" brand of confidence, was a formula for disaster. Adam would no doubt experience this shift in approach more as an abandonment than as an act of love and assurance, which was what accounted for his shaky reaction. It wasn't until Mr. and Mrs. Freer began watching over him a bit more closely—assuring him that he *could* manage his personal hygiene and his school responsibilities, and congratulating him when he accomplished these things—that Adam started to calm down and feel more secure. With this, they reclaimed a sense that they could manage their son, and Tom reclaimed a sense that he could still be helpful to children and parents.

Although there are clear steps that therapists can take to manage helpful conversations that inspire change, the measure of success is in how our comments are construed by family members. Even when we think we've been empowering in our approach, our clients may think otherwise. Whether therapeutic conversations create narrative solutions depends upon how our clients interpret, incorporate, and extrapolate our words to their own lives. Change comes when our conversations affect *their* conversations, and when our reconstructions alter *their* views and actions.

—8—

Retelling Children's Stories, Part I

COMFORT, FIT, AND HIERARCHY

Believe it or not, a decade ago in family therapy, *hierarchy* wasn't a dirty word. According to Jay Haley, hierarchical confusion was the greatest source of difficulty between children and their parents (Haley, 1976, 1980). The hierarchy in therapy consisted of a therapist-in-charge, who directed parents who were not in charge to reclaim their leadership over their children, who were often too much in charge. Thus, therapy restored hierarchical order to families who had lost it.

Salvador Minuchin (1974) referred to parents as the "executive subsystem," thus underscoring their authority *over* their children. It was the therapist's job to strengthen the executive system and to reinforce hierarchical boundaries. Perhaps it was Minuchin's commanding presence that also led therapists to believe that the job called for an authoritative therapist, a directive director.

The structural family therapist's forceful style might now appear confrontational in contrast with the conversational, nonimpositional stance of the narrative therapist. Although the narrative solutions approach is gentler and less impositional, much of our work with children and adolescents does involve helping to shore up the resources of parents so that they reclaim their stewardship of the family. This generally includes purposefully guiding the conversation so that parents change what they do with their children. And we use our influence, albeit differently, to strengthen the parents' influence over their children's lives. So, what's so new? Why all the fuss with these newfangled social constructionist concepts?

A key difference between structural family therapy approaches and the narrative solutions approach is that we look at family structure and hierarchy not as fixed, static, or permanent, but as fluid and evolving. This dynamic formulation of family structure is more than postmodern posturing. It has practical implications for how we converse with children, their parents, and others about the presenting problem.

Consider, for example, a common scenario: parents and children who arrive at our offices locked in a struggle for power and control. The parents may be struggling to assert their authority and make their child behave, while their child resists and defies them. As the problem intensifies, parents may throw up their hands and/or engage adult authorities external to the family. For example, when we first talked with Rachel and her mother, we found a mother who was deferring to relatives, teachers, principals, lawyers, and therapists; a daughter who was defying all adult authority; and a family structure on the verge of collapse. Family Court had assumed an executive position in the family hierarchy; a judge, then a stranger to the family, was about to rule on whether Rachel's mother or a whole new set of adults at an unknown residential facility would take charge of Rachel's future. Certainly, to a structural family therapist, this looked like a malfunctioning hierarchy. Yet, order was restored by talking with family members about how this troublesome arrangement came about in the first place.

The therapist didn't shift sides in this hierarchical struggle (as described by Minuchin & Fishman, 1981), or push for the mother to regain command of her daughter, or arrange that external authorities back off (as described by Haley, 1980). Instead, the therapist questioned mother and daughter as to how the current family structure moved from a preferred to a nonpreferred form. The therapeutic conversation focused on how events evolved over time, and how the current relationship arrangement took shape. Through this process of curious inquiry, we learned that the present "structure" didn't at all represent the preferences of the people who shaped it. After family members were helped to recapture their strengths and understand each other's positive intentions, a more workable structure took its place.

Looking at family structure as evolving rather than fixed allows the therapist not to push so hard. We needn't feel compelled to force an enmeshed family structure to become disengaged or to push a disengaged family structure to become more enmeshed. Instead, we may simply, gently, bring people back to viewing each other in ways that sustained a more helpful structure in the first place and provide them with an alternative explanation for the evolution of their seemingly fixed entanglements. This approach can free them to seek out more suitable options. Family members themselves will then create relationship arrangements that fit with who they wish to be, and that permit them to change that "structure" as they grow and negotiate new life transitions.

With regard to hierarchy and power in parent–child relationships, we make two assumptions. First, we assume that parents and other adult caretakers *are* in a position of having more power and influence than children in the relationship. Appreciating this difference promotes the idea that adults must be thoughtful about, and accountable for, the effects their actions have on children. To ignore this hierarchical distinction is to promote abdication of adult responsibility for children's well-being.

The second assumption is that children need caretaking, guidance, and leadership from adults. Adults are responsible to use their authority to promote, among other things, children's safety, sense of security, confidence, and independence. In the chapters that follow, we'll offer examples of how parents use their guidance and leadership to help children of various ages and at different stages in their development to overcome problems. Obviously, for children to thrive, parents must gauge the extent to which children need their direction, and when children can manage on their own. As we present examples of work with families, we'll discuss some of the factors parents need to consider in making these decisions at various stages in the family life cycle.

Because our goal is to empower parents, let's consider what parents have been through by the time they reach our office. By the time parents call to arrange help for their children, how are they likely to view themselves as parents? How might they feel? How might their views of themselves as parents shape how they see their children? Placing ourselves in the position of the parent seeking help allows us to start the conversation with them empathetically and respectfully.

"YOU DON'T KNOW WHAT WE'VE BEEN THROUGH"

When parents at their wits end say to a therapist, "You don't know what we've been through," they're usually right. They come in confused and overwhelmed, worried by their child's anxieties, worn out from sleepless nights of calming her nightmares, frustrated at their child's seeming lack of concern for defecating in his pants, or possibly furious by their child's opposition, lack of cooperation, and apparent selfishness in the face of their own generosity and self-sacrifice. If their own frustrating experience didn't wear parents down and cause them to question their competence, all the well-meaning advice and thinly veiled criticism they've received certainly has.

Recently, Tom began working with 6-year-old Jed Innis, referred for school phobia. Jed's mother called from her son's pediatrician's office to make the first appointment. The pediatrician had already called and asked Tom to see Jed as soon as he could. When Tom met with Ms. Innis the next day, she said she was unsure of what to do next. She described how Jed had difficulty separating from her when she went to work for the first time early in the summer. At first, she took a strong stand: She left the sitter's house with Jed in tears on two occasions, assuring him that he would be fine. The result was that Jed, in fact, did manage this early separation comfortably. Shortly before the start of his first full day of attendance in kindergarten, however, Jed woke up at 11:00 at night crying, screaming, and in the grip of a nightmare in which his mother had died. The morning of Jed's first day of kindergarten was fraught with tears and pleas to stay home. It was only by way of Ms. Innis' calm resolve that he somehow got to school that day. Jed's teacher reported that he was fine after 10 minutes of crying. Following this early success, Jed's behavior escalated to complaints of stomachaches, then tantrums followed by his mother's wrestling him into the school. When Tom asked Ms. Innis how her efforts were working, she described how she eventually gave up this insistent approach. She then broke into deep sobbing. She spoke of how she started to talk with Jed about the possibility of going to another school, and how she kept him home from school on the day before the first appointment to see his pediatrician.

The therapist initially met with Ms. Innis individually. Tom highlighted her previous success in assuring Jed that it was okay to leave her and go to school. Tom asked what made her give up the approach that had worked so well to get him to the sitter during the summer and to school more recently. Ms. Innis gave the following explanation.

She said that maybe her husband was right, maybe she wasn't a good parent. She said that this seemed to be the prevailing view of everyone around her and that, obviously, she hadn't helped her son with his fears. When asked who in addition to her husband regarded her as a bad parent, Ms. Innis expressed that the teacher had given her quizzical looks, noting that Jed was fine as soon as *she* left the school each day. Ms. Innis described how on the last day Jed went to school, she struggled and finally got Jed into his classroom, only to encounter his teacher rolling her eyes and looking exasperated. She also described how the school principal sprang out of his office to question her about how things went that morning. After Ms. Innis said that it was still a struggle to get Jed to school, the principal mentioned that Jed's father called. He said that Mr. Innis expressed concern that this problem was still occurring and conveyed anger over "the situation."

Ms. Innis took this to mean that the principal and teacher were in agreement with her husband that she was incompetent. As Ms. Innis began to think this view was correct, her resolve to reassure Jed and get him to school lessened.

The information that emerged in our conversation made it all the more unsettling. Apparently, Ms. Innis had taken Jed and left her husband during the previous spring. The separation took place after numerous incidents of Mr. Innis being physically aggressive toward Ms. Innis in Jed's presence. After moving out, Ms. Innis went to work outside the home for the first time in her life. She did this in the face of Mr. Innis's lack of financial support and his ongoing threat to obtain custody of Jed if she didn't return.

As Tom tracked the onset of Jed's nightmares just prior to the beginning of school, he learned that the nightmares began just after Ms. Innis received a threatening phone call from Jed's father and was in tears in Jed's presence. Fortunately, Tom was able to help Ms. Innis piece together this sequence of events and resume taking charge of her son. First, he had a brief conversation with a well-intentioned teacher and principal about Ms. Innis's worry about their view of her. They began to see that the mother's concern about their view undermined her confidence. This conversation elicited a reassuring phone call from the principal to Ms. Innis and an end to the eye-rolling and looks of exasperation on the part of the teacher. As Ms. Innis saw others seeing her in more preferred ways, the potential for her being helpful to her son increased. Ultimately, Jed did attend school willingly, and Ms. Innis did maintain sole custody of her son.

Ms. Innis had marshaled all her resources to leave an abusive man, to obtain employment, and to support herself and her son on her own. Jed experienced the marital breakup and his mother going off to work for the first time. Mother and son weathered these difficult transitions without the emergence of a problem. When Jed first became anxious, it was in the context of witnessing his mother break down while receiving a threatening phone call from his father. The timing of this phone call was unsettling to Jed, who was about to cross yet another threshold in life, and needed all his mother's support and confidence to do so. Jed was to begin kindergarten the next day. He balked, yet Ms. Innis rallied her resources, despite her upset the evening before, and got him off to school. Her resolve was eventually shaken by the feeling that Jed's teacher and school principal shared her husband's view that she was an incompetent mother. Mr. Innis's idea that people regarded her in negative ways temporarily deterred her from continuing on her competent path.

Being a parent is an impossible job. Under ideal circumstances and with heroic effort, the best of us fail only a little, although we imagine others do it better. Thus, parents are usually hypervigilant, paying close attention to how other people see and judge them. By the time parents reach our offices, their preferred view of themselves as good parents has often come under challenge. Parents don't have to go through Ms. Innis's ordeal to assume that others view them in negative ways. Simply hearing words of advice or disapproval from a highly respected relative, friend, or professional may be enough to shake a parent's confidence. Being told that one needs professional advice or help can be sufficient to undermine a parent's sense of competence. As sensitive as we all are about how we are regarded as parents, there may be no other role in life that is so subject to constant scrutiny, advice, and criticism.

APPEALING TO PARENTS AS EXPERTS

The best way to start the therapeutic conversation with parents is to appeal to them as experts on their own children and engage their help in putting together an explanation for how the problem became a problem. Taking this approach fits with what narrative therapists refer to as a "nonimpositional," "nonhierarchical," "collaborative" therapeutic stance. The therapist is not the all-knowing expert guiding know-nothing parents. Assuming this collaborative stance with parents does more than allow the therapist to be a card-carrying member of the postmodern community. This stance strengthens the family "structure" by reinforcing the parents' leadership. Suggesting that the therapist regard parents as experts on their children isn't to suggest that the therapist play dumb or be less the expert. Parents will not be helped if they feel that in addition to being ineffective in helping their child, they have been ineffective in finding a competent therapist.

The therapist is an expert on children in general, the parents experts on their particular children. The therapist knows what information is needed and how to elicit it from parents and children to unravel the mystery of how the problem evolved. He or she knows how to present relevant information that is helpful to parents. The therapist knows how to bring out the parents' strengths, to draw attention to their own knowledge about what has worked, and to steer them toward potential solutions. The therapist helps parents feel that they are at his or her level of expertise in knowing about their child, as opposed to the therapist appearing to be at their level of confusion and helplessness.

Positioning the therapist and parents as collaborators softens the hierarchy from the child's point of view. The child will begin to see the therapist–parent "subsystem" as a united front, rather than viewing the therapist as presiding over a pair of defeated parents. The child will regard the therapist and parents as cocaptains of an adult team that may come to include others, such as school officials, physicians, probation officers, attorneys, and child-welfare workers.

Children who grow up in a world where parents and other adults are devalued must imagine a shaky future for themselves. But if they see their parents (and other adults) as competent and capable, this will help promote a secure vision of their future.

WHAT PARENTS NEED TO KNOW

Lee Combrinck-Graham (1989) proposes useful ideas about the "biopsychosocial" influence of a child. She states, "We have biological models to explain events within an individual, psychological models to explain events of the individual, and family models to elaborate upon events around the individual" (p. 67). Combrinck-Graham suggests that each of these domains will both shape and be shaped by the relationships between events in the other domains, thus the use of the expression "biopsychosocial influence of a child."

Parents' stories or narratives of who their children are include assumptions about what is "within," "of," and "around" their children. Parents also make assumptions about how these domains affect each other. For example, parents make assumptions about what is within their children in terms of inherent capabilities, such as intelligence, manual dexterity, and athletic ability. They make assumptions about things that might be considered of their children, such as whether their children are likely to be slow to warm up to new situations or whether they jump right in; whether they are likely to acknowledge a need for help, support, or guidance or whether they have such strong preferences to be independent that they would never acknowledge these needs. Parental assumptions about what is within and of their children shape what they do around their children. For example, take parents whose concern is aroused when their third-grade son starts off the year bringing home failing grades, yet the boy insists that he's fine and will do better on the next test. If the parents see him as (1) a bright boy who is capable of managing the work, (2) a boy who has always been clear with them when he needs help, and (3) a boy who responds well to challenges when left to his own devices, the parents might unite and tell him that they know he can handle it. Say, however, these parents make a different assumption. They think that the boy's failure is related to the suspicion that they've had that he inherited the learning disability that plagued the mother's two brothers who, in the absence of any help or support, quit high school. In that case, the parents might act differently. They might, for example, ask their son a number of questions about the difficulty of the work, then tell him not to worry about his failure, and set up a meeting with his teachers.

These different actions might have different effects on the child. How a child construes what parents do helps shape the child's view of his parents' view of him. This construction affects how a child feels, how a child acts, and how a child comes to regard him- or herself. If the boy in our example is bright and capable and does respond well to challenges, he might construe his parents leaving him to his own devices as an indication that they see him as he prefers, and that they have confidence in him. This construction might influence him to try harder. If this same boy sees his parents asking him a lot of questions about the difficulty of the work and setting up a school meeting, he might construe his parents as worried, and as not seeing him as capable. In this case, he might begin to wonder about his own capability, or wonder why his parents would not have confidence in him, and he might question whether he can manage the work. This construction might influence him to stop trying. As the parents observe their son not taking charge of his schoolwork, they might construe this behavior as further evidence that their son has a learning problem, even if he doesn't. The boy's view that his parents don't see him as capable of managing his work might, in turn, reduce the likelihood that he would take charge of his own responsibilities, and foster problem-maintaining interaction around schoolwork. When parents' ideas about what is within, of, and around their children are accurate, they are in a much better position to care for their children.

Parents' assumptions about their children shape their expectations, affect whether they give appropriate support and guidance, and influence whether they act as a unified team. For parents to pull together around solutions, they need to arrive at a clear picture of who their children are, who they prefer to be, where they are developmentally, what they can and cannot handle; how they see the adults around them, how they see the adults seeing them, and how they see their present situation. Once parents have a clear picture of what is within and of their child and understand how interaction around their child is influencing the present problem, they are often quick to unite around what is in the best interest of their child. This solution-oriented behavior occurs when the information about the child is presented to parents in preferred-view terms, that is, when therapists talk to parents in ways that confirm their wish to be good parents.

HOW DO PARENTS GET SO CONFUSED?

Even before parents get inundated with opinions and advice, they are often confused about their child's behavior. In fact, they may have divergent opinions that result in conflicts between themselves about whether particular behaviors should be of concern. The likelihood that parents and children will develop difficulties along the way is partially explained by the sheer number of transitions to be weathered. Almost any "new" event requires parents and children to shift their thinking about self and others and decide how to respond. The vast array of required shifts in both viewing and doing is daunting. We all think of the usual: the birth of a child, talking, walking, toilet training, starting school, the birth of a sibling, entering junior high school, entering adolescence, and leaving home. In addition, it's not uncommon for unpredictable events such as illness or death of a family member, or separation and divorce to occur. Obviously, these major transitions may shake parental expectations. However, even mastery of a simple developmental task such as a child learning to feed or dress, or a "first" time event, such as the child's first sleep over, scary movie or nightmare, can be pivotal. Consider the initially fearful parents of a 5-year-old who are finally comfortable with their son riding on a school bus. Now think of them as they hear their son repeat the disgusting phrase he just learned from his bus mates to describe some sexual activity. Or, consider the first time parents leave their 3-year-old with a new baby-sitter and the child bursts into tears as they are leaving. Each of these seemingly commonplace events can have unsettling effects on parents and children.

Parental confusion is fostered by the difficulty that children have articulating their intentions and stating how they prefer to see themselves. Young children's intentions and preferences are not well formulated and often not well articulated. Although it is safe to assume that young children's intentions are positive and that they would like to be "good kids," this intention is often not noticed by parents when children are acting badly. A young child who isn't performing well in school may not say that he wants to do well, that he feels badly about his schoolwork and lacks confidence. A teenage girl who prefers to see herself as competent and independent isn't likely to let her parents know when she's having trouble saying no to her friends who are encouraging her to stay out late. She may not voice her fears about getting involved with an older, sexually active group for fear that others won't see her as mature and independent. Children also have difficulty talking about unpleasant experiences that are embarrassing or shameful. A boy who prefers to see himself as competent isn't likely to talk about defecating in his pants or wetting his bed.

Thus, parents must be signal decoders. Whereas symptoms are indicators that something is wrong, it's very challenging for parents to figure out what symptoms mean. When confused, parents' decisions about what to do are not only shaped by their views of their children, but also by their own narratives of who they hope to be as parents. Parents' stories about who they are or wish to be as parents are shaped by history, particularly by how they see their own parents as parents and how they feel about their own upbringing. A mother may prefer to be close to her children to avoid making them unhappy, and may take a position against being a disciplinarian in light of her resentment toward her mother, who she felt let her father beat her. A father may want to provide firm discipline because he thinks it was his own father's strong discipline that straightened him out and kept him out of trouble. Parents may have strong preferences to be like an admired parent, or may have sworn to never act like a mean or ineffectual parent. Although these preferences aren't often spoken about, they are likely to become dominant at certain points in time, particularly during transition times when children's behavior and parental expectations change. Parents may develop different views about the nature of "new" behaviors that emerge at a particular transition point and whether these actions represent a problem. Should the parents actually agree that there is a problem, they may still come up with different explanations for the child's difficulty. These competing explanations can become a source of conflict for the parents and create confusion for the child.

Regardless of the assumptions made, the advice given by others, and the individual preferences of parents, few parents define the problem as belonging to the whole family or as based in interactions around the child. Most present the problem as in or of the child. There are several reasons for this initial presentation. The dramatic nature of symptoms that children display, such as severe anxiety, phobias, enuresis, encopresis, and the like, make a convincing statement that the problem belongs to the child. Furthermore, the parents may have been advised of a label for the child's difficulty by a pediatrician or school psychologist. Also, the parents might have been urged to get help for a particular condition by an expert on that condition. Sometimes parents are relieved by this expert diagnostic presentation, as it is a favorable alternative to a vague, floating problem that might not be pinned down or solved. Also, the perspective that the problem belongs to the child often relieves the parents from feeling responsible for creating the problem.

Meeting with children alone creates opportunities in working effectively with families. Suggesting that the problem is a family problem or persuading the parents of the virtues of family therapy may only convince parents even further that they are responsible for causing the child's problem. By meeting with children alone, we avoid creating further upset for parents by implying that they are more to blame than they already feel upon initial contact.

Meeting with children by themselves also allows us to understand how they prefer to be seen and consider their actual intention about their behavior. By talking with children individually, we can gain useful information about how children see their own behavior, how they see significant others, and how they see significant others seeing them. Depending on the child's age or level of comfort in talking with the therapist, this information can be gathered in a variety of ways, including interview, play, drawings and, yes, projective storytelling techniques not often considered part of the family therapist's armamentarium. If we believe information about what is within the child would be helpful, we might employ tools of the child psychologist to gain information about intelligence, developmental levels, academic abilities, and so forth.

Difficulties develop in the meaning context of how children see their parents and how they think their parents see them, and in the action context of behavior around them. Children do best when (1) they see their parents as providing guidance, leadership, and protection; (2) when they see parents as having expectations that are in line with their own capabilities; and (3) when parental expectations aren't too divergent from one another.

Let's look at case examples that illustrate our approach to working with children. The first case shows how serious symptoms can evolve from innocent events, and how quickly parents can respond when they have a sense of what fits best for their children.

THE GIRL WHO WAS AN EXPERT ON THUNDERSTORMS

Karen Ross was 5 years old when her mother called to make an appointment for family therapy. Ms. Ross said that Karen had developed a terrible fear of thunderstorms over the past few months. The Rosses would be awakened nearly every morning with Karen at their bedside, asking whether there would be a thunderstorm that day. She would put up a huge fuss, refusing to leave the house if there were clouds in the sky, refusing to swim in the town pool where the family spent many of their summer days (because you could be struck by lightning), and refusing to be away from family members. The family was deeply concerned that Karen might not manage kindergarten, a situation soon approaching. She was beginning to throw temper tantrums when family members ignored her pleas that they not leave the house during a storm. Karen's three older siblings were rapidly losing patience with her.

When Tom met with Karen alone, she spoke at length about her fear of thunderstorms. She was particularly interested in whether Tom knew anything about thunderstorms. Before he could say much about his expertise, Karen, obviously bright, explained how "thunderstorms produce lightning." She said that people could be killed by lightning and that thunderstorms could occur with little warning. Tom asked how Karen knew so much about thunderstorms. She described how her mother taught her a lot about thunderstorms, and how her older sister had shown her a chart with pictures of different types of clouds, highlighting which ones to worry about if they were in the sky. When asked what she would like to see happen, Karen described how she preferred to be rid of this fear and resume going to the pool and friends' houses. When asked how this fear was affecting other family members, Karen said that her sisters were getting mad at her.

Tom's conversation with the parents revealed a key transitional event. The first signs of trouble occurred shortly after lightning struck a tree near the family's home. This event might not have been so troublesome were it not for people's responses to it. Karen's older siblings began speaking with her about what could have happened if one of them had been near that tree. Karen's parents, who saw her as an intelligent child and preferred to see themselves as educators, launched into a lengthy explanation about thunderstorms and the probabilities of lightning striking people. As Karen's fear intensified, so did her demands for information. The parents saw her seeing them as withholding information and thus increased their efforts to talk about thunderstorms. The more the parents explained, the more Karen asked, and the more everyone talked and talked and talked about thunderstorms.

As Karen refused to engage in previously enjoyable activities, the parents most often attempted to reason with her, then gave in and let her stay home. At other times, they became exasperated and forced her to join family activities. There was an ever-increasing level of upset between parents, between siblings, and within Karen herself. The more family members got upset, the more Karen experienced anxiety.

Tom spoke with Mr. and Ms. Ross about Karen's wish to be rid of fear and return to normal life. He restated what the parents said about problem evolution, noting how Karen's curiosity led her to be more and more interested in thunderstorms. Yet, the more she knew, the more upset she became. The parents said they hadn't thought much about this progression of events. They knew that talking with Karen wasn't satisfying her curiosity, but they hadn't thought about the possibility that talking itself contributed to her worry. Once the parents began thinking along these lines, Tom represented what he gleaned from his individual conversations with Karen about her intentions and views of her predicament. He said that Karen was alert to her surroundings and, naturally, wanted to know how strange things like thunder and lightning worked. She felt that her parents and older siblings expected her to be in charge of figuring out whether there would be thunderstorms and what to do when they occurred. Her intention was to get as much information as she could to make an educated decision. Interestingly, without Tom saying anything further, the parents concluded that perhaps they should change their approach and let Karen know that she didn't need to know any more about thunderstorms, or worry about them.

The second session went as follows:

Ms. Ross: Your idea about the thunderstorms worked.

Lund: My idea?

Ms. Ross: Yes, about telling her that we are in charge of whether she needed to worry about thunderstorms.

Lund: What happened?

Ms. Ross: When she asked if it was going to rain on the first two mornings after our visit last week, I said that parents handle the weather. We'd watch the weather and let her know if there was anything to worry about. We also told the other children not to talk about thunderstorms with her . . . to just change the subject or distract her.

Lund: What did Karen do?

Ms. Ross: At first she got angry, then cried when we wouldn't talk with her about the weather. After a few days, she came to our room in the morning and said, "Is it going to rain?" and I said, "What did I tell you?" She said, "You'll say that parents take care of that and that you'll let me know if I have to worry . . . I'm not going to worry about that anymore."

Lund: And?

Ms. Ross: Well, we kept taking the same approach. When she began fussing about not wanting to leave the house one day when there were clouds, we simply told her there was nothing to worry about. We refused to talk about clouds or the weather and made her get in the car.

LUND: How did that work?

Ms. Ross: Fine, she's swimming in the pool again, and she doesn't ask about thunderstorms while we're there.

Karen's parents made an insightful leap. The therapist merely talked about Karen's concern about being in charge of thunderstorms. He did not suggest that the parents' waffling about whether Karen should be required to participate in family activities contributed to her anxiety. As mentioned, once parents explain their children's predicaments differently, they often come up with their own ideas about what to do. Karen's parents not only stopped talking about the details of thunderstorms with their daughter and reassured her that they were in charge of worry about thunderstorms, but they were also calm, clear, and consistent in insisting that she participate in family activities.

As with the Ross family, the goal in most cases with symptomatic young children is to help parents understand what would constitute a helpful conversation with their children and motivate them to have such conversations. Karen felt that her parents were not taking charge of a rather worrisome matter. Similar anxieties develop when youngsters become embroiled in concern about adult matters, such as household finances, or when they see their own behavior as controlling whether their parents will get along. Once Karen's parents reconstructed the evolution of her symptoms along preferred-view lines, they reframed the current predicament and conversed with Karen differently. As a by-product of these new conversations, Karen's symptoms cleared up over the course of three sessions.

Why didn't we simply tell the parents that they should be more firm with their daughter? Or is that basically what we did? When the family came to us, they were letting Karen stay home when she was afraid. After our contact, they were insisting that she go out with them. Why pursue this inquiry into problem evolution or attempt to understand Karen's view of her circumstances? Why not simply tell the parents to take charge?

By presenting information about Karen and her thoughts of her circumstances, the parents were able to reach a solution without the therapist telling them what to do. This avoids the issue of resistance to advice giving, gives parents a feeling that they solved the problem, and increases their confidence to solve other problems. Parents are often pleased with themselves for having solved a problem without being told what to do by therapists. When Tom called for follow-up 4 weeks later, Ms. Ross spoke with delight about how she and Mr. Ross applied some of their new thinking about Karen to their 4-year-old daughter, Tracy. Tracy was acting upset at bedtime and discussing reasons why she shouldn't have to go to bed before her older siblings. Ms. Ross said that she told Tracy that she didn't need to worry any more about bedtime. Since deciding about bedtime was a parent's job, they wouldn't be discussing this decision at length. Tracy was encouraged to go to bed when the parents asked, or go to bed earlier the next night. Ms. Ross expressed how well this approach worked, and how well both her daughters were doing.

WHEN TRANSITIONS ARE CLEAR
AND INTENTIONS ARE NOT

Karen's parents weren't concerned that her worry about thunderstorms was reflective of a deeper problem "inside" or within her. The Rosses saw Karen as bright and capable and not likely to have difficulty with anxiety. The fear of thunderstorms was viewed as related to the accident of lightning striking a tree. The parents were comfortable that managing that specific fear would be sufficient to help Karen. In many instances, children's symptoms or unusual behavior causes parents to question what is within or of their child. Parents begin to reconsider the child's motives, preferences, and true intentions. This was the case with another 6-year-old named Matt.

Matt and his parents were referred by their family doctor. Mr. and Ms. Davis contacted the doctor at their wits' end. The Davises were clear about the transitional event that preceded the problem, describing Matt as jealous of his 3-year-old brother, Sam, since his brother's birth. They saw this jealousy as having escalated over the past 3 years to the point that Matt was physically aggressive, hitting and pushing his brother to the floor daily. On one noteworthy occasion, he threw Sam across the room. Matt's father witnessed this event when he charged into the room after hearing his younger son's pleas for help. On another occasion, Ms. Davis was concerned that her sons were playing a bit too quietly, only to find that Matt had gagged his brother and was in the process of tying him up with a rope. The parents were beside themselves and felt they could no longer allow Matt near his brother unsupervised. Also, there were worrisome reports from school that Matt was becoming withdrawn, disinterested, and not completing his schoolwork.

Tom met with Matt alone to understand what was happening from his point of view. Through this conversation, Matt's preferences, intentions, and worries became quite clear. However, it wasn't Tom's brilliant inquiry with Matt that unveiled Matt's inner concerns, but

Matt's questioning of Tom. The first 15 minutes of the initial session consisted of Matt looking at Tom suspiciously and ignoring questions about what he liked to do. He finally looked at Tom and said, "When are we going to talk about it?"

LUND: Talk about what?

MATT: You know.

LUND: What do you think we're going to talk about, Matt?

MATT: Me. I'm bad.

LUND: You are?

MATT: (*looking surprised and a bit exasperated*) Yes.

LUND: You think you're bad?

MATT: I am bad.

LUND: How do you know that?

MATT: I do bad things to my brother.

LUND: I don't think that means you're bad.

MATT: (*looking more puzzled*) It doesn't?

LUND: No.

MATT: That isn't what Mom says.

LUND: What does your mom say?

MATT: Mom says I used to be good, but now I'm bad.

LUND: Do you like what you do to your brother?

MATT: No.

LUND: Why is that?

MATT: Because it's bad.

LUND: Oh, so you don't like doing things that might hurt your brother, and you don't like Mom thinking that you might be bad.

MATT: No, I don't.

Tom and Matt went on to discuss what happened when Matt did things to his brother Sam that his parents got upset about. Matt rattled off various negative effects, including his parents upset, his feeling bad, and so on. Matt explained that his brother always got him in trouble. He described a recent incident in which Sam sat in a chair that he coveted at the dinner table. Sam smirked, giving Matt the impression that he was rubbing Matt's nose in his victory. Matt's response was to pull Sam off of the chair, eliciting upset from Dad and an even broader grin from Sam, who remained in the desired chair. Matt described several situations in which his brother succeeded in looking good while Matt looked bad to his parents. Looking bad in the eyes of everyone around him fueled Matt's attempts to get back at his brother, which only led to more of the same aggressive interaction. Matt's intentions—which were to be "good," to not hurt his brother, and to not have his parents upset at him and think of him as bad—were not being realized.

Tom spoke with Mr. and Ms. Davis while Matt played in the waiting room. The parents described how Matt was an easygoing baby boy until his brother was born and things began to change.

LUND: What were the first things you noticed?

MR. DAVIS: Matt started crying easily and seemed to want more attention.

MS. DAVIS: We gave him a lot of attention. We expected him to be jealous so we were careful.

LUND: What kinds of things did you do to be careful?

MS. DAVIS: One thing was that we included him with everything we did with Sam. He held him a lot . . . he helped me feed him.

LUND: When did you first get concerned about Matt's behavior?

MS. DAVIS: He started getting rough with Sam. First it was playing rough . . . when Sam was just learning to walk . . . I started getting worried.

LUND: What did you do?

MS. DAVIS: We talked to him about it. We explained that he was being rough and could hurt Sam. I don't think he realized he could hurt him. I don't think he meant to be mean at first.

LUND: How did he respond?

MS. DAVIS: Sometimes pretty well . . . other times I'd hold my breath.

LUND: (*looking at Mr. Davis*) What do you think of all of this?

MR. DAVIS: I think my wife's account is accurate. We worry, though, that he is intentionally mean. He seems to want to hurt Sam. That's the part I don't get.

LUND: That he would actually want to hurt him?

MR. DAVIS: I don't like to think that, but we're worried.

MS. DAVIS: He really seemed to get mean over the last 6 or 8 months

. . . angry at his brother for no reason. I ask him why he is angry. He doesn't answer. I think it's jealousy.

MR. DAVIS: I spent more time with him. We've been careful not to punish him.

As Matt became rougher and meaner with his brother, the parents, for fear that it would increase jealousy and make Matt feel bad, didn't set limits for Matt's behavior. As Matt continued to act in upsetting ways toward his brother, his parents became upset themselves about Matt's intentions and whether he really wanted to be mean. Matt's view was that his mother began to regard him as bad. This view contradicted Matt's preferred view and inspired more aggression toward his brother. Further conversation with the parents was geared toward informing them of their son's actual intentions and deciphering how the problem evolved.

LUND: You really tried to help Matt not be jealous of his brother . . . You've been very sensitive to that . . . went out of your way to include him in caring for Sam. He was an easygoing guy, who, in spite of your attempts, seems to have become angry and jealous of his brother.

MR. DAVIS: That's about how we see it.

LUND: You know he did speak pretty openly with me.

MS. DAVIS: I'm surprised. He said he wasn't talking to anybody. I told him it was very important that he speak with you.

LUND: Well that must have had an impact, because he did it on his own terms. He was pretty clear about what he wanted to talk about. He spoke a lot about his worry that he's a bad boy.

MS. DAVIS: You think he's worried that he's bad?

LUND: That's not exactly what you see at home?

MS. DAVIS: You really think that he's worried about that?

LUND: Yes, but he doesn't exactly act in a way that suggests it. I can certainly see where it doesn't look that way. Actually, I got the sense that his worry that people see him as bad and his brother as good has something to do with his behavior toward his brother.

MS. DAVIS: I don't think I've helped much.

LUND: How's that?

MS. DAVIS: I've said things like, "Do you like being bad?" I guess I hoped he would realize that he was acting badly and do something about it. He didn't seem to care.

MR. DAVIS: If he's worried about being bad, why doesn't he stop?

LUND: That's a good question. He seems to be taking a different approach, one that only sinks him in deeper. From what you've said about Matt's behavior since his brother was born, he's had trouble acting in ways he'd like. It seems that he always wanted to help with his brother and be involved, but as he got rough with his brother and you pointed out that he was, he couldn't really stop himself on his own. Now he seems to be saying that he's upset that people see his brother as good and him as bad. He has no hope of changing that, so he just lets loose with his brother.

MS. DAVIS: So his worry about being bad and his brother being good makes him more jealous?

LUND: It looks that way.

MR. DAVIS: I wonder if we shouldn't have been firmer with him.

LUND: Why?

MR. DAVIS: Well, maybe we let him act rough, and he couldn't stop himself. We were worried about disciplining him, because we felt it would add to his jealousy.

LUND: Is this a new thought for you folks?

MS. DAVIS: Actually, no. At first we did draw a line for Matt's behavior. My sister and my mother went nuts.

MR. DAVIS: She's not exaggerating.

MS. DAVIS: They kept warning us that he would be jealous and angry.

LUND: You let him do things that didn't feel right to you?

MS. DAVIS: I think we did. People really got us worried about this jealousy business.

Apparently, the parents did initially discipline Matt and felt comfortable with this approach. However, the perception of criticism from Ms. Davis's sister and mother caused them to change their approach. This new information contributed to our understanding of the evolving problem. (See Figure 8.1.)

The parents' explanation for Matt's aggressive behavior was that it was motivated by jealousy. The Davises assumed if they gave Matt more reassurance by spending time with him, and if they included Matt in caring for his younger brother, his jealousy might subside and

The Evolving Problem

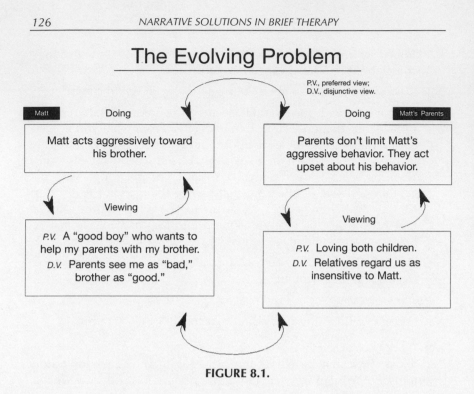

FIGURE 8.1.

his behavior improve. This was a reasonable assumption if Matt were able to manage the situation on his own. As the parents became upset with Matt, as Matt viewed his parents as upset, then viewed them as thinking of him as bad, Matt's aggressive behavior escalated. Matt managed his distress by attempting to get back at his brother, which caused his parents to further doubt his good intentions. They began to believe that Matt was a bad boy.

Armed with a new view that Matt was worried that they thought he was bad, the Davises stopped using that word and instead commented when Matt did positive things. Finding positive accomplishments wasn't a difficult task. Matt was always quick to take on responsibilities at home and did well in school, even though he had been distracted recently. The parents decided to set limits on Matt's behavior with his brother. Interestingly, they felt relieved that they could now do what they always wanted to do when Matt first became rough with Sam, but didn't do for fear that it would contribute to his jealousy. With a different story of the evolution of Matt's jealousy and a new understanding of Matt's inner intentions, the parents set about their mission.

Over the course of seven sessions during a 10-week period, there was a dramatic improvement in Matt's behavior. The results confirmed for the Davises that Matt did have good intentions. His behavior toward his brother improved, and he seemed happier, even though for the first few weeks he spent a fair amount of time in his room for acting aggressively toward Sam.

CONVERSATIONAL SOLUTIONS

In the case of Matt Davis and his parents, the therapist conducted a conversation with a 6-year-old boy and learned about his positive intentions. Matt said that his parents thought of him as bad, and he didn't like it. He didn't like it that they were upset with him, or that they viewed his younger brother as good and him as bad. The therapist circulated this information about Matt's distress to his parents. The Davises realized that Matt was experiencing a gap between who he'd like to be and who he thought he was in the eyes of his parents. The parents altered their approach to Matt and closed this troublesome gap.

The key to Matt's transformation wasn't mere punishment. Limit setting was an approach the parents employed to emphasize that they were not going to allow Matt to treat his brother badly. This approach also helped him be who he wanted to be. Although punishment may have inhibited Matt's aggressive behavior toward his brother, his view of himself and the manner in which he thought his parents viewed him may well have stayed the same. Reminding Matt that he was seen as good, and reassuring him that his parents would set limits to help him act in line with his preferred view, changed his self-construction *and* his behavior.

Thus, the solution to Matt's behavior problem was embedded in new conversations within the family that helped Matt fulfill his true intentions. These new conversations altered a story of Matt that was in the process of being written. This story could have become part of a book in which the chapters that followed consisted of further episodes of aggressive behavior at home and school. As these episodes repeated, Matt might have become increasingly convinced that badness was part of his permanent character, and so would his parents and other adults.[1] Instead, this story in the life of Matt Davis became part of a fleeting chapter in which a boy, once jealous of his younger brother, was helped by his parents to be the responsible person he wanted to be.

[1]For an example of how irresponsible behavior evolved from childhood into adolescence, see the case of Butch Anderson (Chapter 15). In this case, a lack of parental limit setting, along with recurrent family conversations, which reminded Butch that he was seen as the spitting image of his wayward biological father, led to the development of aggressive behavior in a 19-year-old.

—9—

Retelling Children's Stories, Part II

A s we've mentioned, one of the reasons families run into difficulties with young children has to do with the sheer number of
transitions to be weathered. In the cases discussed so far, the
transitional events that kicked off problems were clear to parents. Although this clarity alone didn't lead to their figuring out what to do to
help their children, having some understanding of the context for
symptom development helped to orient their thinking about their children. Often symptoms appear out of nowhere, leaving parents totally
in the dark about the nature of their children's distress.

UNRAVELING MYSTERY TRANSITIONS

Emily Miller was 9 years old. Mr. and Ms. Miller described her as an
excellent student, assertive and confident with other children and
adults. Ms. Miller had an excellent reputation as a teacher of troubled
children. Mr. Miller was a respected college professor, and little brother Andy was as sociable and successful in school as Emily, although a
bit more reserved. Suddenly, from the parents' point of view, Emily
started complaining of headaches and anxiety and having trouble
sleeping at night. Mom and Dad were bringing Emily to school together as much as their work schedules permitted. They tried to reassure
her that she would be okay there. Mr. and Ms. Miller seemed to be doing all the right things, as if they had just read a book on structural
family therapy with a postmodern touch. Yet, even on days when both
parents brought her to school, Emily would cry in class, put her head
on her desk, and end up in the nurse's office. She began putting up a
huge fuss about going to school. At the same time that Emily was ex-

periencing all this anxiety, her mother noticed another, more subtle change in her behavior. Not only was she adamant about school refusal, but she was also challenging her mother about family decisions. Emily's parents had no idea why Emily suddenly developed such troublesome symptoms. In the absence of an explanation, the parents interpreted the anxiety as "within" Emily. They had no sense of how to approach the situation other than by continuing to insist that she go to school and possibly take medication for her symptoms.

In their first telephone contact, Ms. Miller mentioned that she heard Tom's name from the school psychologists at her own school as well as her daughter's. She explained that she and her husband were eager to get help for Emily, although Emily was dead set against the idea of therapy. No one in the family had sought professional help before. Emily's teacher, school nurse, and pediatrician were in agreement with the parents about getting Emily to school each day and felt the parents' firm reassurance was appropriate. It seemed that Mr. and Ms. Miller were being seen by each other and by those outside the family in preferred ways. Their distress derived from confusion and worry about their daughter. The parents' common goal was to relieve Emily's anxiety, have her go to school willingly, stay in class without crying, and return to her bouncy, spunky, good-student self.

When Emily and her parents appeared at the office, Tom asked Emily if he could speak with her alone. Emily made no attempt to conceal her irritation about having to speak with a psychologist. She glared at her parents as Tom introduced himself and grumbled "Mo-o-om" in a low voice as she walked up the stairs to the office. Emily sat stiffly in her chair. She was pleasant, yet clearly unhappy about being there.

LUND: You don't seem very happy to be here.

EMILY: I don't need to talk to a psychologist.

LUND: Who thinks you do?

EMILY: My parents.

LUND: Did they tell you why?

EMILY: Because I didn't want to go to school . . . now I do.

LUND: Your mom mentioned that you missed some school . . . you didn't go because you didn't want to?

EMILY: I was sick. I had headaches. Now I'm fine.

LUND: When did things get better?

EMILY: What do you mean?

LUND: (*thinking that he had an opportunity to compliment Emily for her independent behavior, to connect with her preferred view, and to have her begin talking openly*) You've gotten yourself to school even though you had headaches and wanted to stay home?

EMILY: I'm going tomorrow. So what?

Tom felt less and less helpful as the conversation progressed. Although Emily remained polite, it was clear she was relishing his defeat. She stood her ground, making sure the therapist wouldn't see her as unable to manage her own business. This conversation with Emily left Tom without a clue about the problem's evolution. He only knew that Emily preferred to be seen as mature and capable, and had no interest in talking with a therapist.

After meeting with Emily, Tom had little of substance to offer the parents. He merely mentioned how impressed he was with Emily's take-charge, "I'm okay" approach to things in the wake of her anxiety. He wondered with the Millers if this confident approach might be getting in the way of her admitting to a problem or giving the adults any hint about what might be troubling her. The parents concurred with Tom's description of Emily's personality and shared stories of her more bubbly expressions of being in charge that predated the problem. Tom puzzled with the parents over what might have thrown Emily off track.

LUND: I wonder if anything changed at school this year?

MS. MILLER: We thought about that. We asked Emily and her teacher . . . she's really bright and capable . . . she gets along very well with her teachers . . . with the other kids.

LUND: Nothing at all was going on at home that you can recall—with any relatives . . . friends . . .

MS. MILLER: No, that's what's so puzzling. You'd think that something must have happened to cause her anxiety and her headaches.

LUND: That is puzzling.

Tom and the parents continued, puzzled, through the first session. Mr. Miller could not make the second session, in which Tom wanted to meet with the parents alone. In this second session, Tom walked Ms. Miller through a series of events—what came first, what followed—in an attempt to unravel the mystery. Taking the stance that a detective tracing clues might assume, Tom brought Emily's mother back to the scene of the first symptoms. "What day of the week was it? What happened 1 day, 2 days before?" Starting with the first signs of symptoms, Tom asked questions that would get Ms. Miller thinking about how things might have looked from Emily's point of view. By having people focus on details that they might have missed, they often recall things that help unravel the mystery of symptom development.

LUND: Emily's first symptoms were?

MS. MILLER: She said she had a headache that bothered her at home and was worse at school. She said she couldn't go to school.

LUND: Then you kept her home. You took her to the pediatrician.

MS. MILLER: He said to keep her home for the day.

LUND: Do you recall what Emily said about this?

MS. MILLER: Not really . . . I think she asked why she was having headaches.

LUND: What did you say?

MS. MILLER: I don't remember. I think I told her we really didn't know, but there was nothing for her to worry about.

LUND: I know I'm asking some pretty detailed questions, but do you recall what happened the next day?

MS. MILLER: I think she went to school, but went to the school nurse for part of her day, then I picked her up early.

LUND: With a headache?

MS. MILLER: Yes, I called the pediatrician, who said to bring her in the next day if she still complained of headaches. It must have been the next day when things got more complicated. Emily was crying in her class for a long time. Her teacher sent her to the nurse's office. When Emily told the nurse that she didn't have a headache, she sat for a bit and then was sent back to class. It probably made some sense to send her back, but Emily started worrying that the nurse didn't believe that she was upset and didn't like her. That was when she began refusing to go to school.

Tom's interest peaked at the mention of a discrepancy between how Emily preferred to be seen and how she experienced the school nurse seeing her. He now had a clue about what was fueling Emily's symptoms and wanted to further examine this clue with Emily's mother.

The conversation continued as Tom tried to zero in on the doing and viewing around the problem. Ms. Miller described how Emily bounced back and forth between home and school as an ever expanding cast of adults made decisions for and about her. Looking at it from Emily's point of view, one could imagine things were rather confusing. She had headaches and stayed home from school one day, with the adults agreeing (something was wrong). Her parents then took her to her pediatrician, who said she could return to school the next day, and her parents agreed (nothing was wrong). Her parents then sent her to school. She complained of headaches, and the teacher sent her to the nurse, who sent her home (something was wrong). Emily complained of a headache again, and her parents sent her to school anyway (nothing was wrong). Emily's teacher sent her to the nurse, who appeared to Emily to be put out and frustrated with her. Now we have confusion about whether the adults are managing Emily's headaches, and we have a girl beginning to worry about how significant others view her. As Tom emphasized how Emily might perceive the teacher and the nurse as upset with her, Ms. Miller mentioned that she, too, had been getting exasperated with Emily and asking her what was wrong with her. Since Emily felt that the adults were totally confused about what she should do, she sought a solution on her own. She stayed home.

The conversation between Tom and Ms. Miller continued.

LUND: This all started with a headache? For days Emily was complaining of headaches. Did she seem worried about her headaches?

Ms. MILLER: She did ask a lot about why she had them. She asks a lot about everything. She likes to be in the know.

LUND: Did she ever have a physical illness that she worried about? I mean, when she was younger?

Ms. MILLER: No, she's always been healthy.

LUND: Did anyone in the family have physical problems in the last few years?

Ms. MILLER: I did, but she never worried about that. That was long before this all started.

LUND: What happened to you.

Ms. MILLER: Bell's palsy. It was horrible. The whole side of my face collapsed. It was scary, but I fully recovered.

LUND: When did it develop?

Ms. MILLER: Last winter. Almost a year ago. I've been recovered for almost 6 months. It went away at the end of the summer.

LUND: This was just before Emily developed her symptoms.

Ms. Miller: Yes. Emily was fine when I had Bell's palsy. Her symptoms developed when things were better.

Tom recalled that along with school anxiety, Emily developed a new behavior pattern that didn't fit with having anxiety. She began challenging her mother's authority. Tom was interested in the possibility that this sassy behavior developed while Ms. Miller was ill.

Lund: You mentioned some things that you thought didn't fit together, how Emily began challenging you about decisions you made.

Ms. Miller: When I told you that Emily started questioning my decisions?

Lund: You said she got pretty testy.

Ms. Miller: That was one of the curious things . . . while she seemed to be so anxious, she also tried to tell me what to do. When to take her to friends' houses, when she should go shopping, and so on. The funny thing about it is that she's usually right, she has good advice . . . she's rather helpful in making decisions.

Lund: You didn't mind?

Ms. Miller: Not at first, but she's been getting more and more disrespectful. She's very insistent that things be a certain way.

Lund: She tries to run your affairs.

Ms. Miller: It's sort of gotten to that.

Lund: What about her father? Does she do this with him?

Ms. Miller: She always has input. He's never been very interested in taking what he calls "her advice." I think she has given up on him.

Lund: She doesn't challenge him much?

Ms. Miller: No, not to where he notices it.

Lund: When did Emily really escalate this challenging-your-decisions business?

Ms. Miller: It probably escalated . . . it was subtle . . . it escalated over the summer when we spent a lot of time together. I was taking her here and there.

Lund: While your Bell's palsy was evident?

Ms. Miller: I think so. Yes. But she got noticeably intense this fall around the time she had trouble going to school.

LUND: So while Emily saw that you were experiencing Bell's palsy, she began to increase her attempts to take over.

MS. MILLER: I'd say so.

LUND: The symptoms you experienced came and went. Was Emily clear what caused them, or why they went away?

MS. MILLER: None of us were exactly.

LUND: She became more interested in taking charge when you had worrisome symptoms.

MS. MILLER: Are you saying that she may have been worried about me and not telling me, but kind of taking over?

LUND: It just seemed coincidental that Emily started increasing her attempts to help you, at least that may have been her intention. You mentioned that she was helpful at first. This all happened around the time you had symptoms. Emily certainly wasn't going to tell you she was worried. That's not how she prefers to see people seeing her.

MS. MILLER: You know, I never thought about her being worried about me, but it fits.

LUND: It's also interesting that she developed headaches, and that it was unclear how they had developed.

MS. MILLER: I never thought about this connection. She may have been worried about my Bell's palsy, but wasn't likely to say that. I don't know if I understand why she would develop headaches though. Do you think it was stress? I could see where she would get worried about headaches, I guess.

LUND: I'm not a physician and wouldn't venture to guess about the headaches. But it would make sense that people not being able to tell her why she had them . . . this with her developing worry that the adults in school weren't seeing her in positive ways . . . could be frightening to her.

MS. MILLER: Well, then I'm asking her what's wrong and what she would like.

LUND: I'm not sure what you mean.

MS. MILLER: Well, when I got stumped, I would ask Emily what was wrong, why she was so upset, when she needs the adults to be telling her . . . sort of.

Finally, the mysterious context for Emily's symptoms became clear. Ms. Miller realized that Emily was worried about her Bell's palsy.

Since Emily's preference was to be a take-charge person, she tried to be helpful to her mother by making decisions well beyond her years. She advised her mother about where she should park at the mall, where she should shop, and what she should buy. She also made it clear to the therapist that she didn't need his help, even if she did have headaches and couldn't get through a school day without seeing the nurse. Having a strong sense of responsibility, Emily never let on that she was anxious about her mother's illness.

Ms. Miller could now see that asking Emily what was wrong implied that Emily was in charge and only fueled her anxiety. The confusion among the adults about whether Emily should stay home or go to school further confirmed Emily's belief that *she* should be in charge. Taking on this level of responsibility added to her anxiety about her mother's illness, but this inner distress wasn't noticeable to the adults around her.

Because Emily wished to see herself as capable and in control of her life, it was unsettling to think that the adults didn't believe her physical symptoms were real and vacillated in their belief about her trustworthiness. Her own vacillation about attending school reflected her wavering confidence in the adults. (See Figure 9.1.)

As Ms. Miller grew clearer about the mysterious evolution of Emily's symptoms, she figured out what to do. She talked things over with her husband and explained what she learned about the roots of Emily's anxiety.

Then the Millers spoke with Emily about her mother's illness, reassuring her that it was gone and would never return. Emily showed some interest but offered no suggestion that she might have worried about her mother. Mr. and Ms. Miller, in an effort to have all the adults appear united to Emily, asked that the teacher and school nurse maintain clear and consistent positions. The parents brought Emily to school and arranged that if she cried or complained of headaches, she would stay in the nurse's office briefly and then return to class. The teacher and nurse were informed of Emily's worry that they were upset with her. Both were quick to respond, being calm and supportive as they stuck to the new plan. The adults, who at one point were contradicting each others' movements and plans, now behaved as a coordinated team.

Ms. Miller, who had been easygoing and allowed Emily to help her make decisions about household matters, decided to act more in charge herself. She listened to Emily's input, but it was clear that Emily's remarks became a minor part of her decision-making process. For example, when Emily instructed her mother where to park at the mall, Ms. Miller ignored Emily's insistence when it escalated to rudeness,

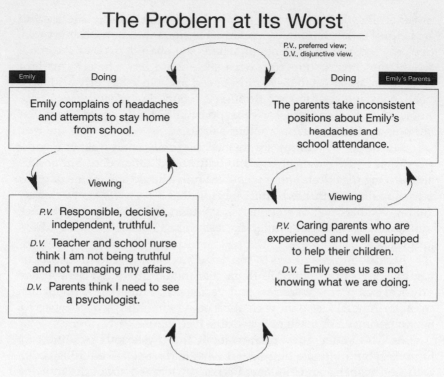

FIGURE 9.1.

asking Emily if she would like to calm down or go home. Emily responded with surprise, but she soon relaxed and enjoyed the shopping trip. When Emily insisted that Ms. Miller pick her up at a friend's house at an exact time, Ms. Miller said that she would make every effort but couldn't guarantee precision. She also assured Emily that she would, in fact, be there. When Emily challenged her, Ms. Miller asked if she would really like to go to her friend's house, because her behavior showed that she wanted to stay at home with a sitter. Emily again calmed down. Emily returned to school and in a matter of 3 weeks was described as her old self. Her headaches also faded away.

The absence of an alternative explanation for curious symptoms can itself trigger problem-maintaining solutions in families. Without an organizing story to explain Emily's anxiety, the parents, pediatrician, and others may have had no other recourse but to see Emily's symptoms as being within Emily, as having a biological basis. In such a case, medication might be considered. Not only would this superficial biological explanation provide little information for the parents to manage the situation, but it would also suggest to Emily that she could not manage her own affairs without medication. One wonders what effect such a decision ultimately might have had on a spunky, bright, and bubbly youngster who wanted to be in charge.

The story of Emily also makes the point that alternative explanations help families weather future difficulties. The therapist had occasion to meet with Emily's mother 1 year later. Ms. Miller described how Emily was having her best school year yet, and that she enjoyed announcing her success to her parents. She then told a story about a revealing conversation she had with Emily's teacher. The teacher expressed concern that Emily liked to raise her hand in class even when she didn't know the answer to questions asked. Ms. Miller explained to the teacher how Emily's enthusiasm about being in charge and showing that she could handle things sometimes backfired. Mom then sat down with Emily and reassured her that she was doing wonderfully in school, but that it was okay if she didn't have the answers to all the questions. She could just relax and not raise her hand. Not only had Emily's symptoms resolved, but also her mother seemed to have latched onto a story about Emily that she carried with her. This story might help Ms. Miller help Emily through the obstacles that crop up for youngsters as they try to grow up and become competent adults.

Thus far, we've described how to help parents unite around an alternative story of the child that explains the problem's evolution. The new story sparks the solution as the parents figure out for themselves what to do differently. There are times, however, when a story is not enough to solve the problem. Specific knowledge about the child's symptoms may need to be incorporated into the story, and specific advice may need to be given that fits within this narrative. When adults lack information about the etiology of complex symptoms that may be biological in nature, they are apt to develop diverging explanations for the problem. These conflicting explanations of what is "in" the child can evolve into problem-maintaining interaction "around" the child, which in turn can lead to psychological difficulties "of" the child. We were taught this integrative lesson by 6-year-old Jeff.

A DISTRACTED BOY

Jeff Carpenter and his parents were referred by his schoolteacher, who viewed Jeff as capable of the work expected of him, yet "in his own world" and forever preoccupied with something other than his schoolwork. He seemed to lose his place while reading aloud. He often didn't follow the teacher's directions or asked for them to be repeated, much to the annoyance of his teacher, who viewed him as disinterested in what was going on in her classroom.

Jeff's father's theory was that his son was much like him, a chip off the old block, who didn't really care for school. His tack was to have Jeff spend time with him in the workshop and at the firehouse, to learn practical skills and downplay the importance of school.

Jeff's mother viewed Jeff as having a strong desire to achieve in school. She viewed him as nervous and unhappy about his marginal success and diminished by his teacher's less than positive view of him. She questioned whether the schoolwork was too challenging for him. The adults' expectations for Jeff were diverging and, although this had not reached crisis proportions, they were beginning to enter into conflict with each other. One day, the teacher pulled Ms. Carpenter aside and suggested that Mr. Carpenter seemed to be influencing Jeff's growing disinterest in school. Mother and father struggled over whether Jeff should stay at home after school and complete work he had not completed in school or go to the firehouse with his father.

As is often the case when there is confusion around a child's learning capabilities, Tom began with a rather standard psychoeducational evaluation of Jeff to ascertain what might be reasonable to expect him to accomplish in school. Jeff appeared to have generally average abilities. He seemed tense and concerned about his performance, requesting constant feedback about how he was doing. Subtle, but striking, was that Jeff seemed to lose his place as he expressed himself verbally. He often looked puzzled and asked the examiner to repeat what he said. This occurred on three occasions in 4 hours of contact. Perhaps because no one had engaged Jeff before in these kinds of tasks in a one-on-one situation, this behavior had never been observed.

Although Jeff's obvious anxiety about his school performance and the clash between parental expectations may have explained his difficulties in part, ignoring the biological in this case would have been disastrous. After completing the psychoeducational evaluation, Tom talked with the Carpenters about what was going on with Jeff. Tom portrayed Jeff as a young man who clearly preferred to succeed in school, but said that his interest in school was being "covered up" by a *confidence problem*. Jeff's confidence had been shaken by frustration over his performance difficulties, and confusion about what the adults expected of him. The people that he most relied on to build a sense of competence (his mother, father, and teacher) all disagreed about what he could and couldn't handle, leaving him confused. Tom noted that the adults' uncertainty about appropriate expectations for Jeff was perfectly understandable, in that an adequate explanation for Jeff's performance problems had not yet been found. In this spirit,

Tom described the lapses in attention he observed and recommended a thorough pediatric neurological exam to explore the possibility that there might be a physiological explanation for Jeff's puzzling attention problems. As it turned out, Jeff's lapses in attention were diagnosed as a mild seizure disorder. When he was placed on an antiseizure medication, things improved.

The knowledge about Jeff's seizures filled in the missing pieces of the story about who Jeff was. Equipped with this new information about why Jeff was struggling in school, the parents were able to unite around similar performance expectations and rebuild Jeff's confidence. Mr. Carpenter supported his wife's efforts to get Jeff to complete his schoolwork, and the teacher and parents stayed in daily contact to monitor his progress. Jeff's enthusiasm for school came out of hiding, and his performance improved.

In the case of Jeff Carpenter, the therapist presented a story of a child that incorporated biological factors into an alternative explanation for his problematic behavior. Jeff was described as a young man who preferred to do well in school, but whose hopes had been stymied by neurologically based problems outside of his control. Two important solutions emerged within this new narrative. Jeff received appropriate medication to control his seizures, *and* the adults changed their interaction around him to bolster his sagging confidence. Neither solution was a "solution" without the other. Simply supplying Jeff with medication to control his seizures, without addressing his worry about his own abilities and the adults' diverging opinions of him, would have been a formula for future confidence and performance problems. A story of Jeff as a "lazy" kid may have solidified. Simply addressing Jeff's confidence problem and altering the adults' interaction around him, without controlling his seizures, would have led to a continuation of Jeff's school problems.

CONCLUSIONS

Perhaps the most important aspect of our approach to working with children is the therapist's responsibility to introduce and cultivate an alternative story for parents of who their children are and prefer to be. Children, through word and deed, do not always inform parents accurately about their positive hopes and intentions. Left to their own interpretations, and influenced by their own narrative of who they hope to be as parents, parents can develop conflicting and unsettling stories about their children. These negative stories can become the "reality" of who the child is and can come to shape the parents' actions around the child. Since young people's stories of self are written largely by their parents, children can arrive at fixed, negative views of themselves that influence their future development and affect how they negotiate the many difficult transitions that face them on their way to adulthood.

Had Matt's parents continued to worry that he had bad intentions, Matt may have seen himself as "bad" and continued to act as such. Had Mr. Carpenter's story of Jeff as a "chip off the old block" who was disinterested in school continued to be reinforced, Jeff may have come to see himself as "stupid" or "lazy" and failed to complete school.

An equally important aspect of working effectively with children is that parents come to see themselves as good parents who can have a positive impact on their youngsters' lives. When parents feel disempowered, defeated, and ineffectual, they often come up with negative and unsettling stories and theories about their children. When parents become reacquainted with their competence and importance to their children, and become equipped with more empowering explanations for how things came to be problematic, they're quick to do what's in the best interest of their children. Power struggles between parents and children subside as parents reconsider who their children are, comprehend their preferences, and reclaim their own influence. New narratives introduced in therapy help parents and children see that their interests aren't mutually exclusive, that they're on the same side, and that they're moving together toward future solutions.

—10—

Listening to the Voices of Adolescents

With young children, we ultimately rely on the parents to be the initiators of new conversations that bring about change—not only to solve the immediate problem, but also to set the stage for the family to move on to the next transition in the life cycle. The therapist serves as an agent, representing the child's wishes and intentions to parents, so that they reconsider their approach to the child.

But children grow older. They develop their own stories of who they are and hope to become. The daunting family transition of adolescence "marks a new definition of the children within the family and of the parents' roles in relation to their children" (Carter & McGoldrick, 1989, p. 17). As children move into adolescence and focus more on the adults they will be, parents tend to see them more as the children they were. Children often prefer to be regarded as independent, capable, and knowing, whereas parents prefer to remain helpful, able to provide guidance, and to be attuned to what their children are going through. Adolescents often act in ways that challenge parents preferences for how they'd like their children to act, for how they'd like to be viewed by their children, and for how they'd like to be regarded as parents by others. "As with clothes and hair styles, roles may be tried on, prized briefly and then discarded or clung to in an attempt to anchor a sense of self. While some of these roles are consistent with family values, they often challenge, if not assault, the mores of the family" (Garcia-Preto, 1989, p. 261).

Michael Nichols (1995) describes how communication between parents and teenagers becomes challenging:

> One reason parents and teenagers have trouble listening to each other is that each side hears the other only as objects in relation to themselves.

When teenagers, who want respect and freedom, come to expect only criticism and control, they shut their ears to what their parents are trying to say and respond reflexively with either resistance or passive compliance. (p. 220)

Although adolescence is a particularly unsettling time for families, this transition can be less difficult when adolescents find their own voices: when they speak up about their own interests and aspirations with the adults around them, and when the adults listen.

MISTAKEN IDENTITIES

It's often difficult for parents to see through their teenagers' rebellious posturing and comprehend their inner desires to become competent and independent. This was the case with the two adolescent girls we've discussed thus far. Rachel asserted her preference to be tough and independent by seeming to ignore her mother's input and getting into fist fights with other girls (Chapter 6); Jean asserted herself by talking back to her father, ignoring his advice, and defying his authority (Chapter 4).

Rachel and Jean's boisterous attempts at self-expression were construed by the adults around them as evidence of failure to mature properly. Rachel's mother wondered whether her daughter might turn out like her father, a criminal behind bars. Jean's father worried that he had lost his loving daughter, whom he had taught to read, ski, play golf, and be feisty and independent. As these caring parents misread their daughters' preferences, they, in turn, came to question their own competence as parents and began acting in ways that seemed out of character. Rachel's mom withdrew as a guide and protector to her daughter, deferring to relatives and outside authorities. Jean's dad battled with his daughter constantly, criticized her motives, argued with his wife over her, and treated her with less respect than he did her brother.

CULTURAL INFLUENCES ON VOICE

It's interesting to speculate how gender stereotypes may have played a role in the evolution of Rachel and Jean's difficulties. They became more rebellious and defiant as they saw the adults around them construe their independent behavior in negative ways. If Rachel and Jean were boys, the first signs of rebellious behavior might have been interpreted by adults as assertions of manhood, feeling their oats, "boys be-ing boys." With more acceptance from the adults, Rachel and Jean may have toned down their escalating attempts to prove that they could manage on their own, without adult guidance. Similarly, if these parents of teenage girls were not thrown by their daughters' newfound defiance to the extent that they changed their ideas about their daughters' intentions, and questioned their own competence as parents, serious problems might not have emerged.

When adolescents' real intentions and hopes aren't being heard by parents, teachers, and other important adults, therapists should spend time with them individually to help them articulate their preferences more clearly. Once preferences are clear, the therapist and adolescent have three choices: The adolescent might decide to change his or her approach to the parents outside of the consulting room; the adolescent and therapist might choose to meet with the parents together to clarify the adolescent's preferences; or the therapist might represent the adolescent's preferences and intentions to the parents. In general, the therapist's job is to help adolescents express themselves in a way that allows parents to understand what they are saying.

In the case of Rachel and Jean, the therapist served more as an interpreter of the young person's voice in conversation with the parents. With permission, the therapist used actual quotes from his individual conversations with the girls designed to help their parents reconsider their motives from a less disjunctive perspective. Once the parents of these teenage girls were helped to recall their own influence in inspiring their daughters' independent spirits, they resumed being the parents they wanted to be. As the parents' voices of influence were strengthened, they began speaking to their children in softer, more convincing tones. Gradually, Rachel and Jean were able to articulate their preferences for independence *and* guidance. Therapy succeeded as these maturing young women and their parents resumed constructive coauthoring of an unfolding narrative, one that contained stories of success, competence, and of acting in line with preferences for all involved.

Rachel and Jean spoke up about wanting to be independent, even though it was in a manner that did not achieve the desired outcome. Unfortunately, many girls who develop symptoms as they grow up are plagued by a difficulty adolescent girls have in our culture in finding and expressing their own ideas and opinions (see Gilligan, 1982).

Carol Gilligan's research indicates that adolescent girls report greater concern about how others view them than do adolescent boys. This finding was supported in research by Shirk (1983), indicating that boys become less other-directed between the ages of 10 and 16, whereas girls do not. Girls also tend to be more concerned than boys with whether people around them are comfortable, happy, and secure. Boys in our culture are apt to be more self-directed. They talk more freely about independent pursuits, competition, material success, and achievement. Since their ideas are supported by the culture, the rebellious behavior of boys may not be construed as problematic. Many adolescent girls, on the other hand, face a dilemma. What do they do when they feel strongly about being their own person, yet perceive their parents as having contrary expectations? How do they reconcile their own preferences when they conflict with the perceived preferences of parents?

Often, adolescent girls reconcile this discrepancy, or disjunction, by submerging their own preferences. They may outwardly defer to the perceived wishes that parents have for them, while they inwardly rage at their loss of self. The emptiness that this dilemma creates is often expressed in difficulties with eating, which, sadly, can be life threatening.

THE EVOLUTION OF BULIMIA IN A 16-YEAR-OLD GIRL

Melissa Stanton's parents contacted their family physician, concerned that their 16-year-old daughter had lost a great deal of weight over the past year. They were alarmed when they discovered that Melissa was regularly vomiting and taking laxatives after eating. In Joe's first session with Melissa and her parents, Mr. and Mrs. Stanton let him know that their inability to help their daughter gain control of her eating problem left them feeling like failures as parents. Although Melissa didn't protest coming to therapy, she did appear put out about talking to a stranger about matters she felt were no one's business but her own. The therapist's impression was that Melissa generally went along with what her parents wanted (except with eating) and that arranging for therapy was yet another example of her parents directing her activities against her will. As Joe conversed with Melissa and her parents, the following story of problem evolution emerged.

Growing up in an achievement-oriented family with two college professors as parents and a younger sister who was an academic whiz, Melissa entered adolescence with a mandate for excellence. She had no doubt about being accepted at a prestigious college and becoming an independent professional, as had her mother. She seemed comfortable that she wasn't a straight-A student and acknowledged that she wasn't as smart as her sister. This modest self-evaluation never got in the way of her ambitions. She'd just work harder if she had to.

Melissa's behavior in early adolescence and her personal construction of her future appeared problem free. She had a circle of friends with similar aspirations, who steered clear of drugs, alcohol, and other common teenage temptations. She participated in a variety of extracurricular activities, including basketball, tennis, music, and ballet, and was attaining the B+ grades she expected to get. From all appearances, Melissa was the teenager every parent wished for. What happened to create a potentially life-threatening problem?

The problem evolved as Melissa found herself working harder and harder to get the grades she expected. It started with earth science. As her parents noticed her struggling and becoming upset with her own performance, Mrs. Stanton encouraged Mr. Stanton, a mathematician, to help Melissa. She also hired a tutor. When English became a struggle, Mrs. Stanton, an English professor, pitched in to help and hired yet another tutor.

As Melissa encountered parents who seemed to think she needed more and more help, her confidence began to wane. Adolescence was supposed to be a time when she would find her own voice, make her own decisions, and determine her own future. Instead, she found that she was having even less say-so about her preferences, hopes, and wishes than when she was a little girl. Being ambitious, Melissa never squawked about her busy schedule or asked for relief from the many activities her parents chose for her. If anything, she intensified her efforts to succeed. Ballet became a struggle. She was not one of the top performers, so she practiced harder. Music came a little easier, but instead of relaxing her efforts, she added the school band to her list of activities.

Melissa's parents were happy to transport her to these various activities and to remind her of her many commitments. Although the parents thought Melissa was pleased, she simply went along with their ideas while giving herself less and less time for eating, relaxing, and considering what *she* would like to do with her time. Noticing Melissa's intense effort in all her activities, the Stantons kept providing and arranging for her to do more.

Because Melissa wanted to be seen as successful in the eyes of her parents, she complied with all the activities they encouraged. She expressed her desire for independence secretly and quietly by attempting to control her intake of food. Her success at controlling eating and at looking thin were reinforced by her ballet friends, who exchanged helpful tips about laxative use. Unfortunately, this "success" at self-control was further supported by the magazines she read and the TV programs she watched, which suggested how girls should look and act.

As the gap grew wider between how Melissa wished to be seen and how she thought she was being regarded by her family, her urge to control and limit her intake of food grew stronger. When Mrs. Stanton finally learned about Melissa's problem with bulimia, she became even more watchful of her daughter's activities. Convinced that her daughter's problem derived from lingering, low self-esteem and her feeling badly that she did not measure up to successful others, Mom persisted in encouraging Melissa's participation in extracurricular activities, and, if anything, became even more worried about her school performance. No time was set aside for family meals, conversation, nurturance, and the enjoyment of food. Rather, family conversations about food drifted more into concerns about Melissa's lack of self-discipline. While Mrs. Stanton tried to resist the urge to search for laxatives or nag Melissa about her eating habits, her fears compelled her to question Melissa about how successful she was in controlling her bulimic urges. These conversations only convinced Melissa further that her mother was more concerned about her outward performance than her inner comfort.

The more Melissa felt controlled by others, the more she tried to control her food intake in a secretive way. As Mrs. Stanton grew more aware of her daughter's bulimia, now carting her to therapy sessions and visits with physicians, along with her many other activities, she viewed herself increasingly as a bad mother who failed to raise a successful, in-control daughter. As the gap widened between how she preferred to be seen (as a good mother who reared a successful daughter) and how she thought she was being seen by others (as a bad mother), Mrs. Stanton's efforts to help her daughter grew more frenetic. The more these helpful efforts were perceived as controlling by Melissa, the less Melissa expressed her wishes for self-comfort and nurturance, and the more vigilant she became about her own eating habits.

Mr. Stanton tried to adopt an objective, scientific approach to this upsetting problem. He probed the literature and learned as much as he could about bulimia. He tried talking to Melissa about what he discovered about the physiological effects of bulimia, but she seemed disinterested. He tried calmly to counsel his wife to back off in her efforts to monitor Melissa's activities. He also talked with her about cutting back Melissa's schedule and possibly terminating ballet. Mrs. Stanton listened, but she stuck to her position. She felt strongly that Melissa loved ballet and would feel defeated by having to give it up. Despite advice from her husband, friends, and physician to limit Melissa's intense schedule, Mrs. Stanton persisted in defending Melissa's gritty determination. She insisted that Melissa could control this oppressive problem if she just put her mind to it. She didn't have to give up any-

The Evolving Problem

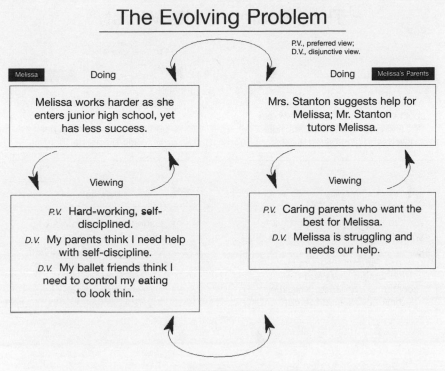

P.V., preferred view;
D.V., disjunctive view.

| Melissa | Doing |
| Melissa works harder as she enters junior high school, yet has less success. |

| Doing | Melissa's Parents |
| Mrs. Stanton suggests help for Melissa; Mr. Stanton tutors Melissa. |

Viewing

P.V. Hard-working, self-disciplined.

D.V. My parents think I need help with self-discipline.

D.V. My ballet friends think I need to control my eating to look thin.

Viewing

P.V. Caring parents who want the best for Melissa.

D.V. Melissa is struggling and needs our help.

FIGURE 10.1.

thing. Advice from family and friends seemed only to fuel Mrs. Stanton's feelings of failure as a parent and drive her to "drive" Melissa. (See Figures 10.1 and 10.2 for a summary of how the problem evolved over time.[1])

MYSTERY QUESTIONS

Having pieced together clues to the evolution of bulimia, Joe posed a mystery question to Melissa and her parents. He wondered, with Melissa, why a young woman with such a fierce sense of determination and independent spirit would require such close monitoring of

[1]Note that while there were differences between the parents in viewpoint, we consider them as a unit for the sake of simplicity. Mr. and Mrs. Stanton shared the same basic preferences. Both felt ineffectual as parents, and Melissa perceived them as more interested in her outward performance than her inner comfort.

The Problem at Its Worst

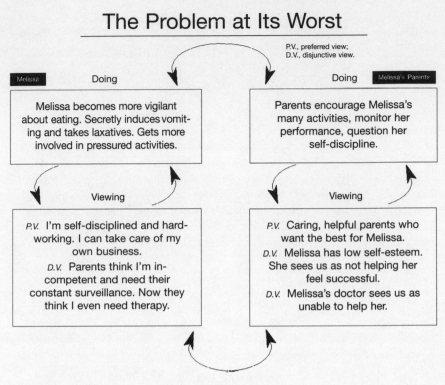

FIGURE 10.2.

her activities. In response, Melissa slowly began to express a preference for managing her own activities and deciding what would be best for her. Still, she hadn't conveyed this preference to her parents, nor had she shown much motivation to change her bingeing and purging habits.

With Melissa's parents, Joe questioned why a young woman with such a strong sense of determination and achievement would fall prey to something that appeared on the surface to be a self-control problem. The goal was to shift the parents' current view of bulimia as a self-control problem to more of a self-nurturance problem. While talking about the preproblem past, Joe and Mr. and Mrs. Stanton discussed the strong sense of responsibility that the parents themselves cultivated in Melissa. He said that Melissa was simply not the kind of person who should have trouble disciplining herself. Surely lack of self-discipline was an inadequate explanation for the emergence of bulimia.

Thus, therapist and family probed for an alternative explanation for this worrisome behavior—one that fit better with the need for encouraging self-expression and self-nurturance. Until the telling of a key story that would take place in the eighth session, Mr. and Mrs. Stanton were still in the dark about what Melissa was up to. Melissa gave them few clues about her inner preferences and intentions. Left to her own interpretive devices, Melissa's mother kept drifting toward the misguided solution of intensely monitoring her activities.

One day, Melissa arrived at Joe's office looking more distressed than usual. Typically, she greeted Joe warmly with a self-effacing smile. Often, when discussing an upsetting event that happened during the week, Melissa's smile evaporated into a stiffened and strained expression. This session began with Melissa's head bowed and her eyes fixed firmly on the floor. Slowly, she began talking in a faint, whispery voice about a funeral she had attended earlier in the day. It soon became clear what was distressing her.

A KEY STORY OF MOTHERS, DAUGHTERS, AND SELF-NURTURANCE

Melissa told Joe that one of her friends from school had lost her mother suddenly in a car accident. Melissa said that the most touching moment at the funeral was her young friend's tear-filled eulogy, delivered from the heart, without any formal preparation. Melissa was impressed that her young friend was able to give voice to her own thoughts and emotions in the presence of all those people. This was something she could never imagine doing. Joe asked Melissa if her parents had attended the funeral. Melissa said her mother had driven her and sat beside her.

Joe then asked whether Melissa and her mom had a chance to talk about the funeral before their session. When he posed this question, Joe couldn't help but think that Melissa would be thinking of her own mother, who was sitting beside her as her young friend spoke, and what it might be like to suddenly lose her at this tender age. Melissa stiffened noticeably. Her face creased in anger as she said that her mother *made* her go back to school to attend her science class, and that there wasn't time for them to talk about anything. Apparently, mother and daughter had sat silently in the car on the way to school and to the appointment, as if nothing had happened that day.

When Joe asked Melissa how she felt about her mom's decision to send her to school that day, she said that she was angry (this seemed an understatement). She said that she was the only student who wasn't permitted to take off from school on the day of the funeral. Although she had envisioned being with her friends huddled together in support of each other, Melissa sat alone in science class, staring out into space.

When Joe asked Melissa if she conveyed her preference to her mother, she replied, "If that's what *she* wanted, what's the point of fighting it? She always gets her way. Why bother?"

Joe invited Melissa to help him understand her mother's motivation. "Why would she make such a decision? Obviously, there was no way you were going to get anything out of science class that day. Were you?"

Melissa explained that because science was her worst subject, her mom was probably afraid that if she missed even one class, she'd fall further behind. When Joe asked Melissa if she herself was worried about missing the class, she said with assurance, "Absolutely not. I have a tutor, anyway. I would have made up the class without a problem. She's right. I *am* doing really poorly in science, but I'll make sure I don't fail. I need to pass to go to college."

When Joe asked if Melissa wanted to go to college, she answered, "Yes, of course I do," looking at him as if he were some kind of dunderhead for implying that there was any other option available.

Based on this conversation with Melissa, it would have been tempting to form an impression of her mother as a cold and heartless person. How could she make her daughter go to school on a day like that, then whisk her off to a therapy session? How could she be so oblivious to her daughter's feelings? When Joe finally got a chance to speak with Mrs. Stanton, a very different image emerged, one more consistent with his previous impressions of her.

Actually, Mrs. Stanton seemed just as upset as Melissa by the funeral. She was equally moved by the young woman's eulogy and her ability to express herself on such a difficult occasion. She became misty-eyed when she recounted how there wasn't a dry eye during the girl's speech, and how nice it was to see the whole community pull together around the grieving family. It was clear that a reassuring conversation with Melissa after the funeral about mothers and daughters, grief and loss, would have done wonders for both Melissa and her mother. But Mrs. Stanton submerged her own emotional needs to help Melissa perform better at science and protect her from the perils of failure. She said that she had a difficult time suggesting that Melissa go to science class (what Melissa regarded as a command, Mom saw as a suggestion), but felt that since Melissa struggled so with science, missing a class would further erode her already fragile self-confidence. Mrs. Stanton, too, wanted Melissa to go to college, to become a successful and independent woman, and failing this required course could hurt her chances. She said that if Melissa had expressed a strong preference to stay with her friends, or said that she was too upset to concentrate on her schoolwork that day, she would have listened and let her stay home from school. Of course, voicing a strong preference wasn't something a bulimic young woman like Melissa was likely to do. Melissa wanted to please others and act as if she could handle most anything that was put on her plate (with the exception of food).

Mrs. Stanton's decision to send her daughter to science class paralleled another recent decision to have Melissa skip two therapy sessions to compete in a basketball tournament. When Mrs. Stanton called to cancel her daughter's appointments, she mentioned how pleased Melissa was to make the basketball team. Her feeling was that to progress in the tournament would bolster Melissa's confidence. Surely, it would be a good thing for Melissa to be with her friends, to be part of a team, and to succeed at something enjoyable. This decision followed on the heels of recent progress. Melissa had gained a few pounds, stopped the self-induced vomiting, and reduced her laxative use. Along with this progress, however, Melissa complained about having to talk about this "disgusting" problem with a therapist when she preferred to have everyone forget about it. Mom figured that she would help Melissa feel more "normal" by emphasizing an accomplishment over an embarrassment. But Melissa's response to the missed therapy sessions, to prioritizing basketball over bulimia, to the renewed emphasis on performance over emotion, was to lose 5 pounds, to increase her laxative use, and move closer to the brink of hospitalization.

This setback was extremely puzzling to Mrs. Stanton, who was trying hard to unravel the mysteries of bulimia. Our thoughts were that Melissa was testing her mother with her complaints about talking to a therapist. She wanted to know where her mom now stood on this key issue of whether how you look on the outside was more important than who you are on the inside. Once again, Melissa perceived that outward appearances won out, even over matters of life and death. It seemed that going to science class was viewed as more important than mourning a tragic death with friends and family, and that basketball took precedence over health-threatening bulimia. Certainly, Mrs. Stanton's intention was not to convey such a grim message, but that was how her recent decisions were interpreted by her daughter who was struggling for selfhood.

At this stage in Melissa's development, her voice wasn't strong enough that she could openly disagree with her mother or speak up about the relative merits of emotional comfort over performance. She was still borrowing her mother's voice, trading off of her view of the world. Instead of speaking up, Melissa did what her mother appeared to prefer—she went to science class. Then, in a silent form of bulimic protest, on the same evening that her friends gathered to comfort each other, she ate a sparse meal all by herself and sneakily took a handful of laxatives to rid herself of all its nutrients. Afterwards, she gave the outward appearance of going to her room to complete her homework, whereas she actually did nothing but stare at the ceiling.

Having talked to Melissa about her actual preferences and intentions, Joe was in a better position to have a helpful conversation with Mrs. Stanton. He began by acting puzzled over the contradiction between how Melissa acted outwardly and how she seemed to feel inwardly about going to science class. He said that Melissa made it clear that the funeral really touched her emotionally, that her mind was still with her friend, her friend's mother, and her own mother while she sat inattentive in class. What Melissa *really* wanted, he said, was to talk with her friends and her mother about their common experience and to receive reassurance, yet she acted as if going to science class was a perfectly fine idea. Joe then asked Mrs. Stanton to help him understand why Melissa didn't speak up about this clear preference to her.

Mrs. Stanton replied that Melissa often did what pleased others, and not what pleased herself. She added that this superficial compliance sometimes disturbed her. She wished Melissa would speak up and tell her what she wanted. If Melissa had done this, she would have altered her decision, which she now realized was not a very good one. What appeared to Melissa as a confident command coming from a controlling mother was actually a shaky suggestion from a confused and worried mother.

Joe and Mrs. Stanton talked about how this tendency to do what pleased others, rather than what nurtured the self, went along with being bulimic. It was out of this discussion that Mrs. Stanton got the idea to try again, to sit down with Melissa and attempt to have the "warm conversation" about the funeral that they had neglected to have before. During their actual conversation, Mrs. Stanton apologized for being so stubborn about the science class. She encouraged Melissa to let her know how she really felt so they could make better decisions together in the future. Mother and daughter comforted each other as they reminisced about the funeral, about the young woman's speech, and about how sad it would be to lose a parent at such a young age. Both admitted that they couldn't possibly speak as eloquently or openly about their own feelings with other people, but wished they could.

This new conversation, which was more about inner preferences than outward appearances, and more about comfort than performance, was followed by a reduction in laxative use and a 4-pound weight gain.

NEW CONVERSATIONS, NEW SOLUTIONS

This new conversation between Melissa and her mother became the springboard for further discussion about the mystery of problem evolution. When Joe agreed with Mrs. Stanton's observation that Melissa was difficult to read and highlighted that it was important for adolescents to articulate their own preferences, Mrs. Stanton seemed relieved. The idea that mothers were supposed to figure out what was going on inside their daughters' heads, without any telltale clues, left Mrs. Stanton with a tremendous feeling of burden. Gradually, Mrs. Stanton became convinced that bulimia was a problem of self-expression rather than a problem of self-control, and she started to talk to Melissa in a way that was more in line with this new perspective.

Mrs. Stanton began having more open-ended conversations with her daughter, in which she expressed interest in Melissa's views and encouraged her to voice her preferences. It was through one of these open-ended conversations that Melissa spoke up about wanting to spend more time with friends, to cut down on her heavy course load, and to let go of ballet (where her laxative use got started). Although Mrs. Stanton invited Melissa to consider the consequences of these decisions, she also conveyed confidence in Melissa's independent judgment. Melissa arranged to meet face-to-face with her somewhat intimidating ballet instructor to explain her reasons for discontinuing dance class. Following this decision to end ballet, Melissa developed a new circle of friends with whom she talked openly about her eating problems. These friends did not encourage laxative use or exchange helpful tips about getting rid of food, but instead encouraged Melissa to take care of herself. In fact, their favorite hangout was a local diner.

Melissa's parents were an invaluable resource in helping bring about change in what appeared an intractable problem. Over the course of therapy, conversations between family members transformed. Most dramatic were the shifts in conversation between mother and daughter. As Melissa made new friends, she fell in love for the first time. For a while, she spent most of her time with her boyfriend, Drew, and ignored her other friends. Although she minimized her eating problems with Drew and told him not to worry about her, Drew worried anyway. Mr. and Mrs. Stanton encouraged the relationship with Drew, who seemed an upstanding young man with a bright future. Suddenly, however, Drew decided he didn't want to see Melissa anymore. The announcement devastated her. At first, she became depressed and stopped eating. This concerned her parents and family physician, who noticed the rapid weight loss. The doctor spoke with Mrs. Stanton about the possibility that bulimia had turned to anorexia and psychiatric depression. He advised that they consult a psychiatrist and consider medication.

Most remarkable were the parents' reactions to these worrisome changes. They stayed calm and supported each other. Mrs. Stanton had a heart-to-heart talk with Melissa about her feelings about the loss of this first love relationship. She expressed compassion for Melissa but also confidence in her ability to weather this blow. Both parents spoke to Melissa matter-of-factly about the physician's concerns. Melissa declared that she wasn't depressed, didn't need medication, and would get over the breakup with Drew in due time. She reassured her parents that she wouldn't let her weight drop so low that she would require hospitalization. The Stantons expressed confidence in Melissa and politely discussed their decision with the physician to continue on their present course with therapy and regular medical checkups.

Melissa's prediction that she would get over the loss of her boyfriend turned out to be accurate. She received a great deal of support from her friends. Melissa's friends began talking with her about their concerns about her eating problems. She considered their input with little resistance. She also talked with her friends and her mother about how Drew was "freaked out" by her bulimia and couldn't handle the responsibility. Melissa simply went about making new friends who were more supportive. Her parents encouraged her resourcefulness.

Melissa and her parents had other noteworthy conversations. Mr. Stanton talked with Melissa about his interest in helping her learn to drive, and Melissa took her father up on his offer. Mr. Stanton's calm, reassuring approach worked well as he guided Melissa to the point that she felt confident taking her driver's test. She passed the test on her first try. The family celebrated by having a pizza party. Melissa ate two slices, one with all kinds of toppings.

Conversations about food also fit within this confidence-building, preference-confirming approach. Mrs. Stanton invited Melissa to eat dinner with the rest of the family and have what she prepared, or she would prepare something else, if she preferred. Even when Melissa's selection of foods seemed peculiar, no one commented. On a few occasions, the family decided to have what Melissa prepared, thus framing her preference for nonfat foods as healthy and strong. Slowly Melissa expanded her eating repertoire, experimenting with different kinds of foods.

At the close of the school year, Melissa decided to attend the annual ballet performance, even though she was no longer a participant. She talked this decision over with her parents, who supported her initiative. The family went to the ballet together, as if to present a united front about Melissa's new life, which didn't include high pressure performances and laxatives. After the ballet, Melissa greeted her friends and instructor and congratulated them on their performance.

Melissa wound up passing science by the skin of her teeth, and her parents congratulated her on her effort. Mrs. Stanton had altered her approach to coaching and prodding Melissa through this difficult subject. She agreed with Melissa that science wasn't her cup of tea and encouraged her to simply pass so that she could take more enjoyable subjects the following year. As Melissa relaxed her expectations, she got through science and focused more attention on the courses she liked and with which she had better success.

In the wake of these shifts in conversation, Melissa gradually gained weight and altered her rigid eating habits. Slowly, she became more comfortable with the weigh-ins at the physician's office, which were indicating that her weight was within a reasonable range for her height and age.

LOOKING TO THE FUTURE

Melissa's parents began feeling more confident that the bulimia problem was under better control, and clear as to how they intended to talk with Melissa so that it stayed under control. Mr. and Mrs. Stanton began to figure out how to steer Melissa through these difficult adolescent years, so that she could become the young adult she wanted to be. Their confidence in themselves as parents was growing stronger. (See Figure 10.3 for a summary of the basic elements of a narrative solution.)

Melissa was heading into her final year of high school. Since the important transition to entering college and leaving her parents home was imminent, everyone agreed it would be a good idea to keep talking. Sessions with Melissa and her parents have continued on a monthly basis.

Melissa now arrives for therapy looking like a different person. She no longer fixes her eyes on the floor, bows her head with shame, or sheepishly hides her face from view. She dresses in a wide range of

A Narrative Solution

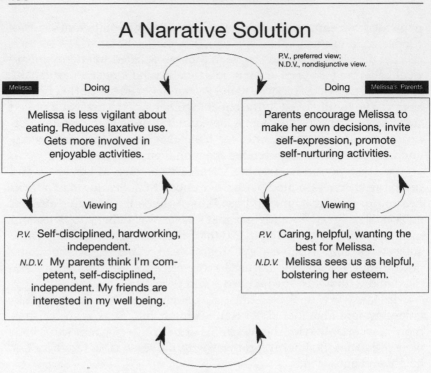

FIGURE 10.3.

colors and brightens while talking about her thoughts and experiences.

Melissa and her parents are negotiating the transition to leaving home successfully. Mr. and Mrs. Stanton talked with their daughter at length about her *preferences* for colleges and helped review applications with her. They have accompanied her on visits to different campuses, and have enjoyed this process of planning the future.

Interestingly, it was Melissa's idea to compose an autobiography and send a portfolio of her work, including essays and creative writing samples, to accompany her applications. Melissa arranged face-to-face interviews with faculty and admissions staff even when such conversations were not required. It seemed important for Melissa to meet people at colleges to help ensure that she'd wind up at a place that suited her.

Recently, Melissa spoke joyfully about her new boyfriend, Alex. She described Alex as someone who was interested in her and her friends, and said she loves their "deep conversations." As she approaches her young adult years, Melissa seems to be figuring out what she wants in intimate relationships with others. She now sees bulimia as a vestige of the past, as a reminder of what can happen if you lose your voice and forget who you are. Melissa's parents feel that they have helped their daughter reclaim her self-confidence and now look to the future with hope.

In their most recent session, Joe and Melissa celebrated Melissa's early admission to a college in New England. A promising picture of the future was beginning to emerge.

As we've described our work with adolescents, we've contrasted cases at the extreme ends of the voice-articulation continuum. At one extreme are the adolescents whose expressions of selfhood are loud, strident, and defiant. At the other extreme are adolescents whose voices are submerged, and whose problems take the form of passive compliance. It's certainly a challenge for parents to interpret and respond to the curious twists and turns of adolescence.

Should parents help children negotiate their teenage years with their own dignity intact and take pride in seeing their children mature and grow confident, consider what they have to look forward to—helping their children leave.

GIVING CREDIT TO PIONEERING THERAPISTS

Before leaving Melissa's story and moving to the next life-cycle transition (young adulthood), let's pause to give credit to the groundbreaking work of Salvador Minuchin. Minuchin opened the eyes of psychotherapists to the influence of family interaction on the life-threatening problem of anorexia and helped hundreds of young women and their families who struggled with these symptoms. The conversations we encourage between young women and their parents follow, in principle, from his pioneering work (see Minuchin, 1974; Minuchin, Rosman, & Baker, 1978).

Minuchin showed that young women suffering these terrible symptoms were trying to become their own persons with their own voices. He brought parents into the therapy room to orchestrate new conversations that confirmed their autonomy. Although the structural approach to change is different from the one we describe, the goals are similar. Without Minuchin's inspirational guidance, we would have had few clues about how and where to steer new conversations between anorexic and bulimic children and their mothers and fathers. In this sense, Minuchin offered a blueprint for the narrative search. We now had a general idea of what stories to look for and highlight that were linked to problem evolution (such as Melissa's story about the funeral), and how to reconstruct the meaning of these stories to promote solutions.

Narrative solutions in cases of bulimia and anorexia emerge when families alter their conversational approach around issues of autonomy. Therapists needn't assume, however, that there's anything wrong with the existing family structure or that overinvolved parents are invested in holding their daughters back from becoming their own persons. Nor must therapists assume that autonomy happens through a process of disengagement from an enmeshed family structure.

In the narrative solutions approach, the tactics for change are perhaps gentler and focused more on forging new connections between family members rather than emphasizing generational boundaries. For example, Melissa initiated more intimate conversations with her mother once Mrs. Stanton encouraged Melissa to talk about her own thoughts, hopes, and intentions. As the Stantons showed interest in who Melissa was on the inside, mother, father, and daughter connected more intimately. They shifted toward a different (self-affirming) involvement with each other, rather than moving toward disengagement.

We would also like to credit the work of narrative therapists Michael White and David Epston, who offer creative alternatives for talking with young women and their parents about matters of selfhood (White & Epston, 1990). White and Epston engage family members in what we would call preferred view confirming conversations. Family members are encouraged to notice the difference between proanorexic and antianorexic conversations and interactions, and to map the influence of these conversations on their lives and relationships. Thus, family members are invited to take a position about whether particular words and deeds have the effect of promoting the power of anorexia or diminishing its influence, and to indicate whether these effects are preferred.

The key difference between White and Epston's approach and our own is that they do not inquire into the mystery of problem evolution. Our interest is in helping families like the Stantons to reconstruct how the self-diminishing problem of bulimia (or anorexia) took shape over time. We then help family members change how they talk with each other so that these symptoms no longer fit within the mosaic of their lives. Within the context of new conversations that promote the articulation of preferences and self-oriented action, problems like bulimia and anorexia lose their stronghold on the young person and symptoms diminish.

━11━

Leaving Parents, Finding Partners: Narrative Solutions with Young Adults

For young adults, the imperative ambition is to establish their own identities, separate from their parents. A critical task for parents is to help their children realize that they can manage their own lives. It's hard to feel like a competent and helpful parent when the task at hand is to let go of parenthood, and it's hard to feel like a competent adult when you haven't quite gotten there yet. Both generations can lose their moorings. Jay Haley (1980) referred to leaving home as the most difficult life-cycle transition that families must negotiate.

Young adulthood is a time when people clarify their own preferences and intentions and attempt to act in line with them. It's a time when we face some of life's great challenges—finishing school, launching careers, and moving out of homes we've lived in our entire lives. When young adults leave home, they begin to create their own cast of characters through love and work. Parents can no longer organize their relationship around parenting when the last child leaves home. They have to draw a fine line between being supportive and helpful, and being intrusive in their children's lives.

CARL LEAVES HOME

When Joe first spoke with him, 21-year-old Carl was living at home with his parents, Miriam and Jake. He said that he had been living

159

with his parents for about a year after dropping out of college for the third time. Carl's parents were pushing for therapy, and they sat right by his side as he nervously dialed the phone to make his first appointment. About 2 weeks before this call, Carl met with the family's physician, Dr. Andrews, also at his parents' urging. Dr. Andrews told the parents that Carl had a panic disorder and recommended that he see a psychologist. The parents then spoke with some close friends, who suggested the Catskill Family Institute.

Over the telephone Joe asked Carl some questions to clarify his views of therapy.

CARL: Hello, Dr. Eron. I'm calling you because my parents think there's a problem.

ERON: Do you agree there's a problem?

CARL: (*sounding shaky*) Yeah. There's definitely a problem. I'm nervous all the time and I can't seem to get moving at all. I just stay in the house.

ERON: What do you think about being in therapy?

CARL: It's really my parents' idea . . . but I guess it's okay.

ERON: Since it's your parents' idea, how do you feel about them coming to the sessions? Do you think they could be helpful?

CARL: I know they'll want to come. They're not sure what to do with me. I know they're really frustrated, and they'll want to talk with you about me.

ERON: Maybe if we all put our heads together we can figure out what these symptoms are about. Would you feel more comfortable talking with me alone at first or with your parents in the room?

CARL: (*hesitating*) I guess I'd rather meet with you by myself, then maybe you can talk with them.

Joe simply could have accepted Carl's statement that it was his parents' decision to seek therapy, then invited the whole family in for the first session. In this case, therapy would have been launched with Carl's voice submerged—not a good beginning to a therapy in which separateness and selfhood were at stake. A simple 5-minute phone call shifted the ambience of therapy from Carl being a passive recipient of help imposed on him by his frustrated parents to Carl being an active agent in stating that there was a problem, that he was agreeable about coming for therapy, that he himself wanted his parents to participate, and that he'd like to tell Joe his own story about the problem without his parents.

In the first session, Carl described recent events in his life. After leaving his third college and moving in with his parents, Carl worked at three different jobs, none of which lasted more than 2 weeks. Each one, he claimed, had something wrong with it. In the first, he didn't get along with his boss; in the second, he had trouble with a coworker; and in the third, they weren't paying him enough for his valuable services. In each instance, Carl complained to his parents about his unhappy lot. They rolled their eyes and in resigned tones that failed to hide their disgust, advised him to try something else that might be more to his liking. Carl lived at home for 1 year and did little but mope around the house during the last 2 months of this time.

Carl complained of anxiety, which he referred to as "shot nerves." It was his shot nerves, he said, that kept him from leaving the confines of his parents' home. Apparently, soon after the third job ended, Carl was out with friends at a restaurant when he had his first and only attack. His heart was pounding rapidly, he was sweating profusely, and he felt like he was about to pass out. He coped with the situation by making up an excuse and hightailing it out of there. His panic subsided as he left the restaurant, but in the car ride home he again felt panicky and pulled over to the side of the road before gathering himself and proceeding home. From this time forward, Carl became leery of leaving the house. He stopped returning phone calls from friends and found a variety of creative excuses for not doing things, work or fun. After a while, his friends stopped calling. Carl's shot nerves rendered him a recluse.

In the second session with Carl, Joe took the time to get a more complete picture of the evolving problem.

A First Attempt at Leaving Home

ERON: Carl, what made you choose a college like Lancaster in the first place?

CARL: It was a small school with a good reputation, not too far from home, but not too close, either. I figured I'd make friends, maybe get on the basketball team. It seemed comfortable.

Eron: So what happened in the friends department?

CARL: I made a couple of friends, but that was about it. I mainly hung out with these two guys, Billy and Sal. Billy was my roommate, and we got along pretty well. But that's all the friends I ever made. It got pretty boring, really.

ERON: You mean you actually got along well with your roommate?

CARL: I guess so. But he and I kind of clung to each other. I never made too many other friends. We just sat around and made fun of the place. You know—the podunk town, the boring classes, the whole bit.

ERON: So what happened to Billy? Did he leave school, too?

CARL: No. He stayed around. I guess he's in his junior year now. I still hear from him. He says it's still pretty boring, but I guess he's happier there than I am here.

ERON: What about grades? How were they when you decided to transfer?

CARL: B's mostly. But in high school I was used to getting A's. I also had a whole lot more friends in high school. I'd go out all the time.

ERON: You were pulling B's, and you had two good buddies, more friends that I can say I had in my first year of college. I remember when I was at the University of Iowa (*pointing to the diploma on the wall*). Lancaster sounds like a major metropolis in comparison. By the time I was where you were in my first semester, I hadn't even met anybody who spoke English. They mostly spoke Iowan out there, and it took me about 3 years to learn the language. I was from New Jersey, and they thought I was some kind of foreigner. (*Carl was now looking at Joe as if he had heard enough of this waltz down memory lane, so Joe wound up his soliloquy.*) I got really homesick in that first year. Did you?

CARL: I called home about once a week and went home for the holidays. That's about it.

ERON: That's funny. I got the impression from your parents that you were having regular conversations over the phone about school and how it was going.

CARL: After I got my first semester grades back, we started talking a lot. I was really disappointed with my grades, and I felt it was time to let them know how unhappy I really was at school. I just wanted to get their advice about what to do. They've always been helpful.

At this point Joe asked Carl to help him understand what these phone conversations back home actually sounded like. If Joe had been eavesdropping, what would he have heard? Carl explained that Joe would have heard a lot of unhappiness and disappointment expressed, which would have built momentum as the conversation went on. Carl might begin by telling his parents how miserable he was at school.

Then, his mother might try to lift his spirits by reassuring him to hang in there. "It'll all be okay in the end," she'd say. At the same time, his father, who never fulfilled his dream to go to college and never got what he really wanted in life, would encourage Carl to get what *he* wanted. "Don't settle for second best," he'd say. "Make sure you go to the right school. Don't compromise your future." This advice would often be followed by a chorus of reminiscences about the past, about how happy Carl was in high school, about how many friends he had back then, and how successful he was academically. Over time, these family chats became more frequent and lasted longer, from once a week to three times a week, from 15 minutes to an hour. The frequent talks culminated in the decision to transfer schools, to try something better. Everyone agreed that the geographic location of the school hadn't really suited Carl. Maybe he'd be happier a little closer to home.

With this, Carl became ambitious and applied to several schools. He finally chose to go to another small school nearby. He had similar complaints about this second school, which he gave even less of a chance than the first. He quickly got into the habit of coming home on weekends and hanging out with his old high school friends who had either gone to the local community college or taken odd jobs and stayed close to home. This time, Carl got the idea that he wasn't being challenged academically or socially, so he applied and was accepted at a "better" school farther away from home. There, he reached the height of his misery. Carl felt panicky before almost every exam he took and had trouble concentrating on his homework. As his grades plummeted, Carl decided to drop tough courses and avoided others by sleeping late and missing them.

With this last go-around at college, Carl tried not to involve his parents in his day-to-day struggle. He called once a week, making it sound like everything was fine. He wanted to tough this one out on his own, prove that he could handle being independent and manage a difficult school worthy of his high intellect. He also figured that he was far enough from home that he wouldn't be tempted to lean on his parents as much. This time the decision to drop out of college came in the form of a sudden announcement rather than a drawn out discussion, and Miriam and Jake were devastated. They expressed anger, even a sense of betrayal. They railed at Carl for concealing his unhappiness and not giving them a chance to help him. In disgust, they allowed that Carl could come home, but insisted that he'd have to work once he got there.

Carl's problem began as he compared life in college to his previous successes and found himself lacking. Carl grew up in a close-knit family, with concerned, loving parents whom he regarded as helpful and always there for him. Naturally he turned to them when he grew doubtful about how he was doing. The frequent, worrisome phone calls weren't always the pattern. The therapist invited Carl to talk about how homesick he was at Lancaster by relating his own story about going away to college. To Joe's surprise, Carl said that he was comfortable being away from home. The worrisome phone calls began with self-doubt as Carl tried to reorient his own expectations for success, to check out whether his then mild concerns had real merit with parents he admired. It was by way of these fretful phone conversations that the problem of panic was born. And it was through these doubt-confirming talks that the idea of failure became more real in Carl's mind. The more real this failure construction became, the more Carl wanted to talk about it.

As Joe listened to Carl's story, the picture of Carl as an ambitious young man contrasted with the image of Carl in his present state: a young man frozen by fear and unable to move beyond the cozy confines of his parents' home.

The Multigenerational Origins of Preferred View

Carl's story offered clues about how to start the conversation with Miriam and Jake. Joe emphasized Carl's past successes in high school, his gumption in applying to so many colleges, and his persistence at trying for something better, even after having what most people would have considered a successful beginning. Then, Joe posed the mystery question. How did a young man with such obvious ambition and talent lose his self-confidence, winding up shaky and unable to get moving?

Contained within the mystery question itself was a reframing of the current problem that now appeared before Mr. and Mrs. Fisher's eyes. Joe deliberately chose not to use terms such as "panic," "panic disorder," "agoraphobia," or "depression" to describe Carl's condition, but instead selected terms such as "ambition" and "lost confidence." Yet, Joe didn't invent these new terms for the strategic sake of twisting the meaning of events in the family, but came upon this language by tracking the course of problem evolution from Carl's point of view. The words that fit Carl's own story had more to do with "ambition gone awry" than "panic disorder." It was within this preferred narrative framework that Joe could now elicit the parents' story.

The story that Jake and Miriam gave Joe about how Carl shifted from confident to timid was informed by their own history—a compelling narrative worth telling. Both Jake and Miriam were first-generation American Jews. Miriam's parents were Holocaust survivors, and much of the rest of her family had been killed in the war. Miriam's father became a highly respected doctor who worked long hours; her mother was a doting yet caring woman who devoted her life to her children and family. Like her own mother, who stayed close to her two daughters after they left home, Miriam hoped to stay close to her two children. Unlike her mother, she developed a career and became a successful part-time accountant.

Jake came from a working-class background. Although Jake's father toiled in the garment district, long hours with little pay, he always fashioned himself an intellectual. Conversant in politics and religion, he'd preside over long conversations around the dinner table, becoming impassioned about the sorry state of the world and offering his enlightened opinions about what would make it better. Jake and his father worked hard to put his two younger brothers through college. Both boys became highly successful men, one a practicing attorney, and the other a physician. Despite the fact that Jake never went to college, he displayed little bitterness about his brothers' achievements. He spoke with pride about his brothers and hoped that his two children would follow their example, rather than his own.

Like his own father, Jake started out in the garment district and through sheer will and determination, became a self-made man, owning his own clothing-store chain and earning more than his two younger brothers. Yet, there were those nagging regrets that Jake passed on in conversations at the family dinner table about never achieving his full potential in life. More than anything, Jake wanted his two children to have what he didn't—a college education.

Alice, Carl's older sister, was now employed as an investment broker for a prestigious firm, had a roomy apartment in Manhattan, a husband, a child on the way, and a brighter future than her parents imagined. But, it was Carl who was the one that Jake felt would soar. He was tall, handsome, popular, well spoken, smarter than smart, and a sure bet in Jake's mind to become the person that Jake was never able to be. Having this sense of narrative history, it was easy to understand the intensity of Jake's current disappointment with Carl.

The Evolution of Panic: The Parents' Account

The tale that Jake and Miriam told of panic building over time dovetailed with Carl's account. They too described Carl as an excellent high school student, popular and confident, and headed for a bright future in college. Jake and Miriam reveled in their son's early successes. They attended all of Carl's basketball games and took pride in his many achievements. As Carl got ready for college, they became intimately involved in the decision-making process. They visited several campuses with Carl and helped him with his many applications. Ultimately, they were pleased with Carl's choice of schools and had every reason to expect he'd be happy there.

Midway through his first year at college, Carl began calling home more often, sounding worried and unsure of himself. This was a new experience for his parents. They were used to talking to a strong, confident son who felt that he could take on the world. As evident from their own histories, Jake and Miriam wanted to see themselves as helpful and giving parents. They hoped to give their two children every opportunity to succeed in life, to expand upon the narrow range of possibilities afforded them by their own harsh early years. When they detected in their usually confident son's voice the disturbing sounds of disappointment, Jake and Miriam responded in a way that befit their preference to be opportunity-giving parents. They joined in Carl's concern and traded ideas with him about other possibilities for success. Unfortunately, their helpful overtures only confirmed Carl's doubts that he was failing to live up to his lofty potential.

At this point in time, Carl began to regard himself as less than successful in his parents' eyes, but he had not run out of steam in his effort to leave home. He continued to experiment with ambition. Jake and Miriam regarded Carl's second attempt at college as being too soft, as not properly challenging his intellect. To counteract this unsettling view, Carl tried for something a bit harder the third time around, applying to a more challenging school farther from home. It was at this large, anonymous school far from home that Carl experienced the first symptoms of anxiety, and in a noble effort *not* to appear soft and weak, he concealed his growing distress from his parents. (See Figure 11.1.)

When Carl finally called to announce that he had dropped out of his third college and was on his way back home, Jake and Miriam were unable to contain their disappointment. It came pouring out in waves.

Family conversations evolved from celebrations of success, in which everyone gazed into the future with hope and optimism, to revelries of regret, in which everyone talked about the past with a sense of longing and loss, and stopped talking about the future with any sense of confidence. Carl was now convinced that he *was* a failure and that his parents saw him that way. Jake and Miriam were now equally certain that they failed to help their talented son reach his full potential in life. (See Figure 11.2.)

At this stage in the conversation, we also had the necessary infor-

The Evolving Problem

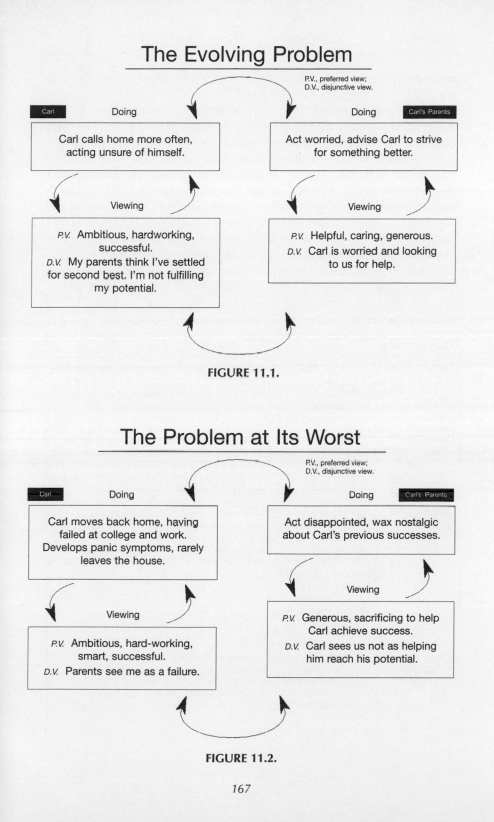

P.V., preferred view;
D.V., disjunctive view.

Carl Doing

Carl calls home more often, acting unsure of himself.

Doing **Carl's Parents**

Act worried, advise Carl to strive for something better.

Viewing

P.V. Ambitious, hardworking, successful.
D.V. My parents think I've settled for second best. I'm not fulfilling my potential.

Viewing

P.V. Helpful, caring, generous.
D.V. Carl is worried and looking to us for help.

FIGURE 11.1.

The Problem at Its Worst

P.V., preferred view;
D.V., disjunctive view.

Carl Doing

Carl moves back home, having failed at college and work. Develops panic symptoms, rarely leaves the house.

Doing **Carl's Parents**

Act disappointed, wax nostalgic about Carl's previous successes.

Viewing

P.V. Ambitious, hard-working, smart, successful.
D.V. Parents see me as a failure.

Viewing

P.V. Generous, sacrificing to help Carl achieve success.
D.V. Carl sees us not as helping him reach his potential.

FIGURE 11.2.

mation to fill out the matrix of views for Carl and his parents (see Figure 11.3).

When people are taking little or no action, it's best to focus on their thoughts rather than their movements. Ambitious young men like Carl, with strong preferences for achievement, are likely to be thinking about action, even when they're not doing anything. Should the therapist fall prey to the trap of suggesting or prescribing new action, the net result might be resistance, stiffened further by the therapist's unwitting challenge to the young adult's preferred view. Carl was now fixed on the idea that his parents regarded him as lazy and unmotivated, and he was more than well attuned to their disappointment about his inactivity. Any hint that the therapist also thought Carl should get moving again would firmly position the therapist alongside Carl's parents in viewing Carl as a disappointment. This was a formula for no new action.

Vantage points	Carl	Miriam	Jake
Preferred view of self	Smart, popular, successful, ambitious, hardworking.	Generous, caring, hardworking. I want Carl to fulfill his potential.	Generous, hardworking. I want Carl to have more opportunities than I had.
View of significant others		Carl seems aimless, lazy, unambitious. **D.V.**—Carl thinks I haven't helped him reach his potential.	Carl seems lazy, aimless, unambitious. He's squandering his potential. **D.V.**—Carl thinks I haven't helped him.
View of family of origin	My mother and father are generous, sacrificing, hardworking. **D.V.**—They view my sister as successful, me as a failure. My grandparents instilled hard work and ambition in my parents.	My parents' dream was to give me every opportunity in life. I want the same for Carl.	My parents weren't able to help me reach my full potential. I want to make sure Carl reaches his potential.
View of therapist or other helpers	My parents think therapy is a good idea. The therapist seems interested in my ideas and preferences.	Therapy seems like a good idea. The therapist thinks I can be helpful to Carl.	I'm willing to give therapy a try. The therapist thinks I can be helpful to Carl.

FIGURE 11.3. Matrix of views.

Here's how the conversation went as Joe tried to remind Carl of the person he once was and still wished to be.

Thinking Action

ERON: I can't believe the effort you put into filling out all those college applications. How many?

CARL: I'd say about 20 between the three times I went to college. I guess that's a lot.

ERON: Twenty, that's amazing. It takes a lot of drive to keep thinking of new options and act on them.

CARL: (*smiling*) From what you're saying, maybe I should have been a little lazier back then. Maybe I'd still be at Lancaster and getting close to graduating. All that ambition didn't help me out a whole lot.

ERON: My sense of people like you, who have really high expectations of themselves, is that they keep thinking ambitious thoughts, even when it looks like they're not doing a whole lot. I wouldn't be surprised if, even after applying to three colleges, you were still thinking of a fourth.

CARL: Well, to tell you the truth, I do still think about it. Lately I've been thinking about going to Dutchess [a local community college] just to get started again. I don't want to say anything to my parents about this. I don't want to get their hopes up again.

ERON: You have a great deal of sensitivity and respect for your parents.

CARL: (*near tears*) I've really put them through a lot you know. They had high hopes for me, and they worked hard to put me through college. They wanted me to have all the opportunities. I've really let them down.

This conversation about Carl's admiration for his family was helpful in setting the stage for Joe's next session with the parents. Joe could now speak with conviction about Carl's high regard for his parents and how his confidence problem was fueled by the nagging idea that he couldn't measure up to them or his sister. Such an explanation would fit with Jake and Miriam's preference to be good parents, yet motivate them to consider other (more empowering) ways of helping their son. Although this was all useful information, Joe and Carl were now squarely in the unsettling realm of how Carl regarded his parents and his sister, and how he viewed them viewing him. The spark that the therapist detected when he and Carl were chatting about Carl's ambition evaporated, and he wanted to get it back. Joe decided to steer the conversation back into Carl's private thoughts about action.

ERON: You really think highly of your parents. You're keeping the ambitious ideas you have to yourself so they don't get their hopes up.

CARL: Yeah. I was thinking of applying to another local college for the next semester but not letting them know about it until it happened. I thought I'd just sign up for a couple of courses, just to get my feet wet again. My parents are planning a trip to the islands to get away for a while. I know they're nervous about leaving me alone in the house. I was thinking I'd let them know about my plans before they leave, just to boost their confidence a bit.

ERON: That sounds like a different approach. Keeping your ambition in check, not letting it run wild like you did in the past. I think you're on to a new strategy.

It's interesting how even when people seem inactive and appear lethargic, they often have creative ideas about possibilities for action. When therapists inquire about these ideas and refrain from imposing their own advice, people speak about hidden ambitions. Carl was thinking privately about how to build his parents' confidence by enrolling in college courses on his own and announcing his new college plans before they went off on vacation. Carl was doing for his parents what the therapist wanted them to do for him (build confidence). The next task was to prepare Jake and Miriam for new action without "spilling the beans" about Carl's plans and help them see that Carl was still looking to them to build *his* confidence.

A Conversation about Building Confidence

MIRIAM: (*looking worried*) We're so frustrated with Carl, we don't know what to do. Should we push him a little? You tell us that he has a confidence problem, and we don't want to hurt his confidence more by pushing too hard.

ERON: In my talks with Carl, what's coming out more and more is that beneath that lazy-looking exterior is an ambitious guy. He just keeps his ambition hidden away, because he doesn't want to disappoint you again. He looks up to both of you for how hard you've worked, how much you've achieved in your own lives, and how much you've given of yourselves. He's got both of you, and Alice, up there on a pedestal, and he feels like he doesn't measure up.

JAKE: It must be tough for him to compare himself to Alice. Alice has done the most with what she has, and Carl hasn't. It's hard for me to think of Carl looking up to us. He's got so much more going for him than we do.

ERON: But Carl knows, like you know, that he hasn't taken full advantage of his abilities. And he feels pretty bad about it all. He feels he's lacking in what you have—determination, stick-to-it-iveness, an ability to finish what you start.

MIRIAM: What do we do to help Carl with his confidence problem?

ERON: If you suggest something for him to do at this point, he'll only get worried about letting you down again. Between you and me, I think Carl's getting ready to try again, and I'm trying to contain my own enthusiasm about directing or advising him—to just let his own ideas take some shape.

MIRIAM: So you don't think we should do anything really. I guess we can wait, but we're getting pretty inpatient with Carl's inactivity.

ERON: I think the real challenge is going to come when Carl does try something again, like a job or school. What do you do when he once again loses confidence in himself and looks to you for guidance?

MIRIAM: I'm not sure what you mean?

ERON: Carl's pattern is that when he gets worried that he's not succeeding at something he sets out to do, he goes to the people he most admires to check things out. He trusts that you will be there to help him, and he values your opinion. He'll look to you to see if you still have confidence in him. The only time he didn't check in with you was at his last school. That's when the panic problem started.

MIRIAM: We've always encouraged him to try something new and different when he gets upset. I don't think that was helpful. Do you, Jake?

JAKE: I guess not. But I don't want to see Carl settle for something beneath his level.

MIRIAM: (*gently to Jake*) I think maybe he just needs to finish something, Jake. Even if it's below his level. Just get "a little success under his belt."

Leaving Home Again

At this point, Joe had met six times with Carl and his parents. Family interaction had changed somewhat. There was less talk of disappointment and less probing and pushing about how to get Carl moving again. Carl began to feel more comfortable socializing. He started to drive short distances to friends' homes, but hesitated about a longer trip one friend wanted to take to New York City. Carl told his friend that he was nervous about driving and being in cars for long periods of time. His friend responded sympathetically, suggesting that they stop along the way, and that he do the driving. Carl took the trip with his friend, felt no reason to stop along the way, and had no experience of panic.

By the 10th session Carl came up with another new plan. He ran it by Joe before breaking the news to his parents. The idea was to go from New York to Virginia with a good friend who had already lined up two jobs handling paperwork for a trucking company. The young men had plans to take an apartment and stay for at least 6 months, from November to May. The job paid pretty well, and Carl hoped to take care of his own expenses without relying on financial help from his parents.

In discussing this plan with his parents, Carl chose to emphasize the part about wanting financial independence. He said he intended to stay at the job for awhile, save some money, and rebuild his confidence about living independently. He explained to his parents that school carried too much of a burden of failure to try again right now. Carl's plan met with an unenthusiastic but generally accepting reception. Miriam endorsed the plan, but reminded Carl that she expected him to stick it out for the whole 6 months. Jake tried his best to contain his disappointment and sought comfort from Miriam about his vanishing hopes for his talented, but aimless, son.

Carl headed for Virginia. Joe left Jake and Miriam with the prediction that Carl would write or call at some point "to express his frustration and check out how he was doing with them." Based on past experience, Joe said, it was safe to assume that Carl's confidence would sag at some point and he'd look to his parents for a boost. While Joe tried to reassure Miriam and Jake about their importance to Carl, they were having trouble seeing themselves that way. They simply crossed their fingers, hoped for the best, and said they'd be in touch.

Sure enough, about 2 months into the new job, Carl called home with the old familiar ring of disappointment in his voice. He said he was bored, that he and his friend weren't getting along all that well, that the truckers he had to work with were "lowlifes," and that he wanted to come back home. Miriam refrained from offering advice. She scheduled a session in which she reviewed with Joe the narrative of the evolving problem. They talked about Carl's confidence problems, his parents' importance to him, the predictability of this latest conversational event, and its significance to Carl's future. Joe reminded Miriam of a helpful comment she made to Jake in one of our sessions. Remember, you said, "I think he needs to get a little success under his belt." Joe suggested that this idea still had meaning. "Since Carl is looking to you for confidence building, you're now in a wonderful position to help him get some success under his belt. Here's an opportunity to reverse an old pattern by reassuring Carl that you and Jake still have faith in him, that you know he can complete what he started."

Miriam left this conversation feeling clear about what to do. She called back to tell Joe that she and Jake did speak to Carl over the telephone. Miriam did most of the talking, but Jake stayed on the line, giving Carl the idea that both parents had confidence in him. She said that their talk went well. Carl agreed that he would go the distance with his disappointing job and remain bored in Virginia until May. At that time, he and his parents would talk about what to do next.

Interestingly, this marked the end of family therapy. New conversations between Carl and his parents were launched at a pivotal time in Carl's life, as he attempted once again to leave home and become the adult he wanted to be. Joe arranged a follow-up session with the family soon after Carl returned from his successful venture in Virginia. At this meeting, it became clear that the reassuring telephone conversation Carl had with his parents when struggling in Virginia revived Carl's confidence and reawakened his ambition. This helpful conversation became a blueprint for future conversations in the family that helped Carl leave home.

Carl called 6 years later to tell Joe that he got "some success under his belt." Over the 6 years since his Virginia trip, Carl completed several ventures. He took on other odd jobs, then landed an attractive job in New York City in the film industry. This success sparked another attempt at college as Carl realized the practical value of a diploma to his future career. Carl now has a diploma, a glamorous job in Manhattan, his own apartment, and a new love relationship. (See Figure 11.4.)

A NARRATIVE SOLUTION TO OBSESSIVE–COMPULSIVE DISORDER

As young adults leave home, a cast of others becomes assembled through friendship, colleagueship, and romance. It's within these new partnerships that problems can develop.

A Narrative Solution

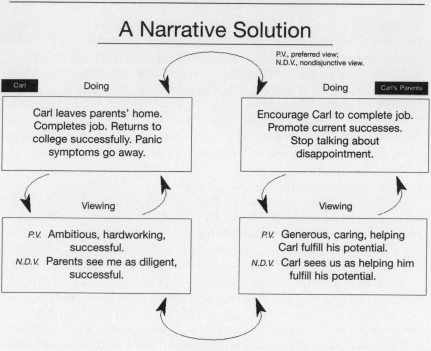

FIGURE 11.4.

Recently Tom received a telephone call from a young woman whose family he had seen several years ago, when her sister was failing at school. Tom had met with Valerie on a few occasions in the family sessions. Valerie, now 22 years old and living with two other young women while she attended college, said she remembered Tom. She called, hoping that he could help her.

VALERIE: Dr. Lund, this is Valerie. Do you remember me?

LUND: Yes, I do.

VALERIE: I'm calling because I need a psychiatrist. Are you a psychiatrist?

LUND: No, I'm a psychologist.

VALERIE: Do you know about OCD [obsessive–compulsive dirsorder]? I need a specialist in OCD.

LUND: Why are you concerned about OCD?

VALERIE: I'm doing all kinds of things. I went to a counselor at school.

He said I have OCD, that I need medication from a psychiatrist (*tears*). Do you know of groups? He said that there are support groups for people who have OCD.

LUND: I can give you the names of some psychiatrists who are very nice and very good. You sound kind of sad about this news the counselor gave you.

VALERIE: I am. I don't want to be a mental patient.

LUND: Are you worried about these things you're doing?

VALERIE: Kind of. They're getting in the way of things.

LUND: And you feel that you would like to pursue medication and support groups?

VALERIE: Not really. I would like to talk to you about it.

LUND: How about if we do what you would like? I'm not a specialist in OCD and I'm not a psychiatrist, but we could figure out what these symptoms are about and what to do from there.

VALERIE: I'd like that.

In this initial telephone conversation, it became clear, even without knowing much about the specific nature of Valerie's symptoms, that the notion that she "had OCD" and that she needed a psychiatrist, medication, and support groups was unsettling. When Tom turned the conversation over to Valerie's preferences, asking her if she would like the name of a psychiatrist or specialist in OCD, she indicated that she wanted to talk about "what these symptoms were about" and to figure out "what to do from there."

By connecting with Valerie's preferences, Tom subtly suggested that Valerie had the power within her to reconsider the meaning of her symptoms and do whatever fit to resolve them. Solutions were possible, whether to seek medication, group therapy, or to resolve the problem through conversation with Tom. In the first session, Tom asked Valerie about her troublesome symptoms.

VALERIE: It's crazy, I'm embarrassed to say. I used to do things in a certain order. Now I have to do things a certain number of times. Now, if I have certain thoughts in certain places, I have to go back and do something again. See, I can't even explain it. Am I crazy?

LUND: How do these things get in the way of you doing what you would like to do?

VALERIE: What do you mean?

LUND: How do they interfere?

VALERIE: I can't study anymore.

LUND: What happens when you try to study?

VALERIE: If I have a certain thought, I have to go back to the beginning of the page and read it over.

LUND: So you do get to know the material?

VALERIE: Yeah, on about two pages. I know the beginning of what I need to study real well. I can't finish studying what I need to.

Valerie went on to describe how her former 10-minute drive to college now took her over 1 hour. If she had certain thoughts as she was driving past certain landmarks, she had to go home and start again. She described numerous other ways in which behaviors that she felt forced to do interfered with all kinds of activities.

LUND: What are the "certain thoughts" that make you start again?

VALERIE: They're horrible.

LUND: Horrible thoughts about what?

VALERIE: They're about someone. They used to be about my mother. Now they're about Mark, my boyfriend . . . actually my fiance! I think Mark is getting tortured or killed. It feels like I don't even mind it. Then I feel terrible, I feel guilty. It's sick. Then somehow if I go back, maybe I can undo it. I don't want anything to happen to Mark. I love him. It's crazy.

LUND: These thoughts creep in about your mother and Mark?

VALERIE: It used to be my mother, now it's Mark.

LUND: When was it about your mother?

VALERIE: When I was 9 or 10.

LUND: How about before that?

VALERIE: It never happened before that. My other counselor thought that the stress of my parents' fights when I was 9 brought out my compulsiveness. I was always pretty organized. I liked things a certain way.

LUND: You first had these thoughts about your mother and they were terrible. You were 9 or 10. Before that you were pretty organized. Was being organized a problem?

VALERIE: No, it actually worked pretty well. I like things neat. I did well in school.

LUND: Then you started having thoughts you didn't like about your mother.

VALERIE: They were horrible! Like she was being tortured or I wanted to torture her. I felt guilty, terrible, worried that something might actually happen to my mother.

LUND: Something might happen because you had bad thoughts?

VALERIE: Yes.

LUND: You didn't want to have bad thoughts about your mother?

VALERIE: No, I wanted to have good thoughts . . . she's my mother.

LUND: How did these bad thoughts affect your mother?

VALERIE: That's a good question. I guess I worried that they would.

LUND: Did you act badly toward your mother?

VALERIE: No.

LUND: I wonder if she knew about your thoughts?

VALERIE: No.

LUND: I wonder why these thoughts crept in when they did. Think there was a reason?

VALERIE: I think so. I hated my parents fighting. I thought my mother started it.

LUND: Did she ever know how you felt?

VALERIE: No. The thoughts I had were so terrible, I wasn't going to tell her.

LUND: You protected her from these thoughts?

VALERIE: Yeah, I guess so. I protected her. I worried something might actually happen to her. Maybe I would do something. She would really hate me.

LUND: Some people would have let their parents have it . . . would have shown a lot of upset toward Mom and Dad.

VALERIE: I don't feel comfortable doing that.

LUND: You protected Mom from these thoughts.

VALERIE: I guess. I like things a certain way. Maybe that's OCD. If I care about Mom and Dad, I shouldn't have bad thoughts.

This conversation brought out a narrative picture of the evolution of symptoms that Valerie now calls OCD. Tom learned from Valerie that the current thoughts that drive her to do "crazy" things that she doesn't want to do were also present when she was only 9 years old. The "horrible" thoughts first occurred when she witnessed her parents' fighting.

Valerie revealed herself to be a person who prefers to be responsible and organized, in control of her feelings, yet caring and sensitive to others. As she witnessed her parents' fights, these preferences came under strain. Valerie "hated" her parents' fighting and blamed her mother for it. Yet, because she preferred to be responsible, caring, and in control of her feelings, Valerie did not express these worrisome thoughts to her parents. She took on full responsibility for having and undoing the bad thoughts, while concealing her personal discomfort from everyone.

The Seeds of a Solution

Interestingly, in this brief excerpt of conversation, Valerie herself began to weave an alternative explanation for the OCD—an explanation that contains the seeds to the future solution. In responding to the mystery of how OCD first interfered with her life at age 9, Valerie reconsidered the meaning of these symptoms. The conversation highlighted Valerie's inclination to protect the other while neglecting the self—recalling the cultural theme of voiceless young women discussed in the last chapter.[1] It's no accident that following Tom's comment about Valerie protecting her mom from knowing her bad thoughts Valerie then says, "Maybe that's OCD. If I care about Mom and Dad, I shouldn't have bad thoughts." Valerie began to explain the evolution of her symptoms in preferred view terms. OCD is now being seen as an outgrowth of caring for others and remaining silent about inner distress. The therapist continued to highlight the theme of "protection of the other."

LUND: If you care for someone, you'll protect them from these feelings.

VALERIE: Not just them, me. I guess I worried that I would be rejected or something. My sister never complained. She didn't seem to notice the fighting.

LUND: So when you have bad thoughts about someone you care about, you might do some things to get rid of these thoughts.

---

[1]Once again, we see a practical application of Carol Gilligan's research on the dominant other-orientation of young girls. As she suggests, the inclination of young women to lose their voices in the wake of strong sensitivity to the comforts of others is best restoried and reframed as a developmental strength.

VALERIE: I undo them.

LUND: How did you undo them when you were 9?

VALERIE: I used to have to get in and out of bed about a million times ... I didn't get any sleep. If I had a bad thought when I laid down, I had to get up and turn on the light, take my doll out of a drawer, put her in another drawer, turn off the light, and jump back in bed before I had a bad thought ... about a million times ... I never got any sleep.

As the conversation progressed, Valerie described how her symptoms disappeared when her parents' conflicts quieted down, about a year later. She never spoke with her mother or father about how she felt and continued to have symptoms until her parents got along better. This discussion of the curious origins of symptoms situated OCD in a narrative context. We gained insight into the evolution of her current situation. The therapist shifted the focus to more recent times. He began by emphasizing Valerie's preference to be organized and in control—the competent side of OCD.

LUND: You really didn't have symptoms for more than 10 years?

VALERIE: That depends on what you mean by symptoms. I like things a certain way. I get pretty tense when things are disorganized. Isn't that part of OCD?

LUND: Would you have called me if things were as they were a year ago?

VALERIE: No.

LUND: Why not?

VALERIE: Because I didn't have these thoughts and compulsions.

LUND: You kind of like being organized.

VALERIE: Yes (*laughs*), I do. Like I said, it helps me in school. I still get A's in everything.

LUND: Even with all of these troublesome thoughts, things you have to do ... with all of the trouble studying?

VALERIE: Yes, I'm pretty determined.

LUND: Valerie, this organization and wanting things a certain way sounds like something you like and something you're always going to want to do.

VALERIE: But I have to get rid of these obsessions and compulsions.

LUND: That's for sure. Do you know when they started again?

VALERIE: Not exactly.

LUND: You said that you were troubled by thoughts about your boyfriend [Mark].

VALERIE: Yeah.

LUND: Did anything happen in your relationship?

VALERIE: I think that these thoughts have to do with stress. They got worse when he went away . . . to college.

Valerie identified key strengths—determination, self-discipline, organization, success at school. She also integrated past and present. OCD originated in her upset over her parents' conflicts in the past and was rekindled by her distress over her boyfriend's moving away. Valerie acted like a codetective, piecing together the clues to problem evolution and resolution. She'd started to think that OCD may be linked to how she handles her distress over the actions of others. This theme is explored further.

LUND: The bad thoughts started when Mark went away?

VALERIE: No.

LUND: When he began talking about going away?

VALERIE: I'm not really sure.

After more discussion:

LUND: Have you been upset with him at all?

VALERIE: What do you mean?

LUND: Well, you said that these symptoms came up previously when you were upset with your parents arguing. So I thought maybe . . . ?

VALERIE: I was upset with him last summer.

LUND: Why?

VALERIE: Well, that's over. He gets upset when I mention it. I don't talk about it much.

LUND: Mark doesn't like you talking about it?

VALERIE: He says I don't trust him. He gets upset. He worries that I will cheat on him. That's what happened. He went out with another girl last summer, and I didn't know it. I found out from a friend.

He kept denying it. Now he writes me, saying that I probably will go out with someone.

LUND: Did you tell Mark how you felt?

VALERIE: I tried. He's not a very good listener. He said that I probably wanted to do the same thing to him. But I didn't. I told him that.

LUND: Wait a minute. You're telling Mark how you feel about him cheating on you and he looks for reassurance from you?

VALERIE: Yes. I felt bad for him.

LUND: You felt bad for him after he cheated on you!

VALERIE: Yes.

At this stage in the conversation, an alternative explanation for OCD was under consideration, namely, when you have bad thoughts about someone you care about, you might do compulsive things to get rid of these thoughts. Valerie began to see that her approach to managing upset with Mark resembled what she did in the past when she worried about her parents' fighting. Mark was cheating on Valerie, and she was uncomfortable about *his* behavior. Instead of voicing *her* discomfort and transferring the responsibility for irresponsible behavior over to Mark, Valerie conveniently (for Mark) experienced bad thoughts and heaped all the responsibility onto herself for undoing these thoughts. The absurd extremes to which Valerie had taken her nurturing of others' sensitivities became more obvious. Restorying the past lead Valerie to reframe the present situation and open possibilities for new action.

Valerie became *determined* to keep history from repeating itself. She had a frank talk with Mark about her discomfort with his behavior. She let him know that if she can't have confidence in his fidelity, he can kiss other women all he wants, but he can also kiss their relationship good-bye. Valerie is now using her determination in a positive, self-confirming, solution-oriented way, rather than a symptom-producing way. Acting in line with controlling her own discomfort, rather than trying to control emotions, helps Valerie to feel more in control. The bad thoughts and compulsions gradually diminish. She resumes doing the ordinary things that her symptoms once blocked her from doing.

The Client Explains

The next conversational segment is a transcript of the fifth and final session in which Valerie reviews her progress with Tom and offers her own explanation of what worked to make things better. Typical of this approach, you'll see that Valerie credits herself for change, not the therapist. The therapist is seen in Rogerian-like terms as someone who reflected her thoughts, took interest in her views, and validated her feeling that she was okay. Fittingly, Valerie, once preoccupied with the wants and needs of others, now finds strength and *power within* herself to reconstruct her life and move on to the future with confidence.

In the ensuing transcript of the final session, we underline those portions of dialogue that demonstrate how Valerie restories and reframes the meaning of her symptoms in ways that confirm preferred views of self. These preferred-view reconstructions of the past, present, and future are the basis for the rapid resolution of complex symptoms, often called OCD. We include much of Valerie's commentary, because her analysis of her own dramatic transformation provides clues to what works in therapy.

LUND: Thank you for allowing me to videotape our conversation.

VALERIE: That's okay. This might be interesting. How should we start?

LUND: Maybe you could mention why you first called me.

VALERIE: Well, I had a lot of obsessions. I felt guilty a lot of times, and to reduce guilt, I would perform these rituals. I couldn't get to sleep at night because if I had a bad thought on one part of the road, I would have to drive through that place again, and if I didn't do that before midnight, I could never remove that awful thought.

LUND: It might be there forever.

VALERIE: Yes, it would be there, and I would be uncomfortable forever, and that would be the worst thing that could happen. I was worried that I would need medication, but it was at a point where I would do anything.

LUND: People labeled this OCD and suggested that you needed medication.

VALERIE: Yes, a sickness you could never get rid of. It did not respond well to drugs or to therapy. I didn't want to seek help, because I didn't want to be told, "You are a psychiatric case, and there is nothing we can do for you." I took a chance and came here, and I think it is working, for the most part.

LUND: I was impressed with all of the things you noticed about how these troublesome symptoms evolved, how they affected you and what you did to solve this.

VALERIE: I'd be driving down the road before midnight, at 11:55, rush back before a deadline, and it was like I was forced to make everything alright. I couldn't concentrate on schoolwork. I couldn't sleep. I couldn't even have a conversation.

LUND: Things have changed.

VALERIE: I actually read the newspaper all the way through today. I didn't have any problem reading today.

LUND: You would have had trouble before this?

VALERIE: A month ago, I couldn't read the newspaper.

LUND: You also just mentioned trouble driving.

VALERIE: A few weeks ago every time I'd drive somewhere, I'd have to go back where I started. Now I'm getting places on time. I think more clearly.

LUND: How about sleeping?

VALERIE: Better. Actually I would even have compulsions in my dreams. For the last 2 weeks I haven't. You think about this during the day, but you would hope that when you went to sleep, you wouldn't have to think about it. You never get a rest.

LUND: You know you never mentioned these things happening after you went to sleep.

VALERIE: Well, now I'm having nightmares. I never had them before . . . people being killed, pretty horrible things. I didn't think I had any reason to have nightmares. I guess because the guilt I associated with bad thoughts was taken care of through compulsions, I didn't need to have nightmares. (*laughs*) So maybe this is a good sign . . . to actually have natural guilt and fear and do what everybody else does . . . have actual nightmares (*laughs*) which is better than having to walk back and forth or having to drive around a bunch of times.

LUND: (*laughing with Valerie*) So it's a good trade-off.

VALERIE: Yes, it's much better. I would love to have a nightmare instead of that other stuff. Besides, I don't think they'll last.

LUND: So you think that if you have angry feelings toward people you care about, you could have nightmares right now to work them out, but soon you'll just have these feelings, and they will be just how you feel.

VALERIE: I had a recent nightmare . . . something happened to my parents. I woke up . . . maybe I was relieved that I could have these thoughts, that I didn't need to undo them with compulsions. My parents were still there in the morning.

LUND: So having these thoughts didn't really do anything to anybody.

VALERIE: Dreams are a way for releasing your fears. They're okay for now . . . they're refreshing. I used to have good dreams but a bad time when I was awake.

LUND: The nightmares seem like a temporary alternative to undoing these thoughts during the day. But soon you won't need nightmares, either. You've come to look at things differently. You said last time we met that "I'm not trying to pretend. I'm not trying to create my own reality in my head about things. It's okay for me to have feelings about people I care about that are much less than positive."

VALERIE: Before I started coming here . . . these compulsions were a way of suppressing my feelings about people . . . about my parents before, and more recently about my boyfriend. My whole life was suppressed. Like with my parents, I thought that if I have bad thoughts . . . well . . . I couldn't tell them . . . well . . . I couldn't even have them. I thought they liked my sister better, because I was mad because they were fighting. She always seemed good and happy. If I was mad at them, they would reject me, and I felt guilt anyway so I had to suppress these thoughts. If I expressed my feelings, I was afraid to . . . I was afraid to get mad. With Mark, things weren't working out for us. I couldn't admit that things weren't going as they should. No matter what happened, we should act like a couple. I couldn't even have negative feelings.

LUND: You seem to be interested in experiencing and expressing your feelings.

VALERIE: I shouldn't have thought like that in the first place. Coming here, I almost have to reconstruct my whole life because it was so . . . I would make up everything that I wanted to be true. Now I have reality . . . which isn't so much fun . . . but I guess its the only way I'm going to deal with my life . . . if I actually face reality.

LUND: You've said that things have changed since you came here, yet I don't think I've done very much. Have you noticed that.

VALERIE: Yeah, you've been reflecting what I say.

LUND: It seems like you've figured this all out, and I just went along with you.

VALERIE: Well, I did it. I think, because you listened and know something about this. I figured it out. You haven't been telling me how to look at it . . . but you backed up what I was thinking. I think I understand why I was doing these things. It makes sense. I had a misconstrued concept of why I was having these compulsions. I needed someone to say, "No, there's not something wrong with you." I had a totally misconstrued concept. I figured out how I thought obsessions and compulsions kept me and people I cared for protected. If I had bad thoughts, my mother won't be protected . . . something will happen to her. I was angry at her and I didn't know how to deal with it. I couldn't talk to anyone. I would have to deal with it myself. I felt so guilty about these thoughts . . . I had to do compulsions to protect people. I remember that you said you noticed how important it seemed to me to protect people. I thought about that and realized that this was the basis of my obsessions. I think that really was the problem. I protect other people and torture myself.

Now I see that. It was almost easier to beat myself over the head than to say, Mark, I don't like what you are doing. I didn't want to risk hurting him or losing him or causing a big rift in the relationship. It was easier to make up a reality that I had upsetting thoughts about him because I didn't drive or walk a certain way.

LUND: You seem to like this idea of dealing with this new reality.

VALERIE: I was getting so obsessive. I thought my relationships hinged on whether I did these great acts of courage or protection to earn the right to be with that person, who was treating me badly anyway. Now I see that there is no relationship between me doing compulsive things, undoing these thoughts, and how we get along. Maybe I thought I couldn't face problems in our relationship. It was almost easier to torture myself and hope the thoughts would go away than to deal with them.

LUND: You started to speak more about how you felt and what you would like in your relationship with Mark, rather than protect Mark by not talking.

VALERIE: I would like to be protected for a change. Instead of having to worry about everybody else. I almost feel uncomfortable if I'm looked after too much. That is going to change. I'm taking care of me. (*laughs*) I don't think I am asking for anything unreasonable, really. I wouldn't mind being looked after.

LUND: You're going to let people around you know that. Can they handle it?

VALERIE: It is reasonable . . . they should. <u>I wasn't really opening my mouth to tell Mark how I want to be treated. I would let him do what he wanted and deny my feelings. I should be more demanding . . . push a little for what I want. Maybe he would listen. I'm going to get the guts to speak up for what I want</u>.

LUND: Has it been a <u>lack of guts? It seems to me that it took a great deal of courage and strength to be as protective as you've been and to manage these feelings on your own. Now you feel less obligated to be protective, more free to speak up.</u>

VALERIE: <u>I guess it has taken courage or strength to protect everyone else. I do feel more free to speak up for what I want and for how I feel.</u>

A narrative solution emerged out of a series of five helpful conversations between a therapist and a young adult in distress. Over the course of these conversations, Valerie restoried the evolution of her OCD symptoms in a way that fit the adult person she wanted to be.

First, she talked about the effects of OCD on her current life and took a position against OCD and its power over her. Then, she recalled the emergence of these negative symptoms in her past life and remembered the context within which they developed. She reclaimed her positive intention to be an in-control person who could figure out how these awful symptoms had taken over her life, so that she could do things differently in the present and future. She realized that her preference to care for others and to be sensitive to their emotional needs rather than her own had gotten in the way of her taking control of her own life and steering its course. With this preferred view-confirming explanation for symptomatic behavior, Valerie decided to engage in a new conversation with Mark that ultimately altered her symptoms.

Tom was fortunate to have contact with Valerie 3 years after their final session. She expressed that she ended the relationship with Mark and proudly talked about her new relationship with another man who she said "loves me and trusts me like he does." Valerie was completing college and in the process of applying to graduate schools, free of symptoms of OCD.

CONCLUSIONS

In this chapter, we've described therapeutic conversations with a young man and a young woman. The young man developed symptoms as he tried to leave home. The young woman developed symptoms as she fell in love and considered marriage. In each case the young adult was helped to counter the influence of dominant cultural expectations.

The conversations with Carl and his parents cultivated statements of preference that lay outside the dominant cultural narrative for young men (see Gilligan, 1982). Carl was helped to reconcile his unbridled ambition (a dominant male aspiration) with a need for comfort and reassurance (a less dominant male aspiration). His sensitivities toward others—how he viewed them and how he thought they viewed him—were brought to the forefront, permitting his parents to see that he still needed their guidance and confidence building. Carl's desire to achieve and become successful (preferences that men often talk about) was coupled with his preference to be sensitive to his parents, worthy in their eyes, and receive their guidance (preferences that men don't often talk about). Interestingly, once these comfort–reassurance–guidance and other-oriented components of Carl's life story were emphasized, he was better able to become the successful, independent man he wished to be.

One of the culturally dominant themes for young women is to cast aside their own preferences and aspirations in the interest of being helpful, caring, and sensitive to others. For Valerie, submerging her own preferences was the basis of her symptoms. Valerie was helped to reconcile her wish to be sensitive to others with her desire to be successful, independent, and self-oriented.

Both preferences were regarded as strengths. Once the self-oriented aspects of Valerie's preferred narrative were highlighted, she talked with her partner in a way that helped her feel in control of their future relationship. She also regained confidence that she could complete college and achieve her career goals without the interference of OCD.

—12—

The Power of Untold Stories: The Case of Sammy's Secret

Adults who wind up in our offices often feel they've failed to succeed in love and work, accomplishments they think should already have been realized. They may still be struggling to complete their education, establish a career, form a meaningful partnership, or have children. They may still be attempting to conduct their lives in ways similar to or different from their own parents, yet failing to reach their aspirations.

As adults, they may be following in footsteps they don't want to follow in—having a distant marriage like their parents, being stuck in a humdrum job like Father, overwhelmed with household responsibilities like Mother, addicted to drugs or alcohol like a wayward parent, or having violent arguments with a spouse like they saw their own parents do. Or, they may be departing from traditions that they hoped to maintain—having conflict in a marriage when their own parents never fought, struggling in a career when their parents were successful, or experiencing behavior problems with children when their parents had firm control.

As Sam grew older, he had many of these concerns. "Sammy" was what they called him when he was younger. Now he preferred just plain "Sam." He was 28 years old when he first came for therapy. Now, he's 35 and he and Joe are still talking. Sam and Joe have now met about 60 times over a span of 7 years. There have been stretches of time when they didn't meet at all for well over a year. Sam came back when he reexperienced old symptoms or when he was tackling a life transition that reminded him of his secret—or what once was his secret.

At the time Sam called to arrange his first appointment, he was vague about the nature of his concern. He said he wasn't sure about where he was heading in life. In the first session, Joe tried to get a better sense of what Sam meant when he said he wasn't sure about his future.

ERON: Sam, you said over the phone that you weren't too sure where you were heading in life. Can you help me understand what you're not sure about?

SAM: My dad is talking about retirement, and he wants me to take over the family business.

ERON: Is it a good business?

SAM: Yeah. The business makes a lot of money, and I know it really well. I've been working with him in the hardware store since I was 12 years old. I've got some good ideas about where to take the business so it can be even better.

ERON: It sounds like a nice opportunity.

SAM: It is. But my father's a pain. He's tight with money, and I know he's gonna have a hard time letting me do things my way.

ERON: What would be your way?

SAM: I care more about people than money. I feel like we need to hire some new people, good reliable people, and expand the business.

ERON: Sounds like you want to do things differently from your father. How do you like to deal with people?

SAM: I like to get to know customers personally. And I like to treat the employees with respect and get to know them too.

ERON: And your dad?

SAM: He doesn't want to part with his money. He never takes vacations. He has a successful business, but he doesn't ever enjoy his life. He takes no interest in the people that work for him, and he's tight about giving them time off or even giving them praise for their effort. I just pray I never end up like him.

ERON: Is that one of your concerns? If you take over the business, you might start acting like your father, even though you don't want to?

SAM: No, not really. I know I'll never do things his way. I guess it's just these few years between now and when he finally really leaves the business. That's what I'm worried about.

Sam and the therapist focus on Sam's concerns about "where he's heading in life." He doesn't want to be like his father and is considering how to deal with the impending shift from working for his father to running the business himself.

When Joe asked Sam if his father acted differently outside of the business, Sam described how distant his father had always been. He'd had a serious drinking problem when Sam was a young child. At that time, Sam viewed him as critical and insensitive toward him, his mother, brother, and sister. He said that his mother's approach to his father's drinking and cantankerous behavior was to preserve at all costs an illusion of stability and security in the family. Over the years, Sam's father stopped drinking, yet there was never any discussion between parents and children about this event. Sam and his siblings did talk about their upset over their father's drinking privately and tried to support each other around it. Sam felt that these conversations were helpful.

The contradictions in Sam's presentation were glaring. Joe spent 45 minutes talking to a 6'3", imposing looking 28-year-old man who greeted him in the waiting room with a firm handshake, as if they were about to engage in a high-powered business meeting. Then, when they arrived at the consulting room, Sam described with supreme confidence how he planned to run the next 5 years of his life after taking over the family business from his father. He was clear about how he viewed his father and spelled out how he wanted to be different from his father.

CONVERSATIONAL POSSIBILITIES

There were several conversational paths to pursue at this juncture, and some were more likely to be helpful than others. An MRI therapist might ask for a more specific behavioral definition of what appeared a vague complaint. For example, the therapist might ask Sam how he'd know that he was heading in the right direction in life. What would be the telltale signs of progress? What would he be *doing differently* in the future that would give him the idea that he was on the proper course? Whereas such questions might unveil a clearer complaint, they also might not move Sam off his fixed spot. Sam might continue to focus narrowly on the world of work and talk about how he pictured himself functioning in the future as the sole proprietor of his business.

A more confrontational approach would be to challenge Sam about his tangential ramblings and suggest that it was time to get down to the real business of talking about real problems. Of course, such a conversational strategy was even more likely to bring about resistance, in that the therapist would be suggesting that he knew more than the client knew about his "real" problem.

A third approach would be to address the mystery of these curious contradictions. Since Sam viewed the therapist as someone who could help him plan his future, *and* since Sam appeared more competent in the domain of business planning than the therapist felt, this curiosity seemed worthy of comment. With Columbo-like puzzlement, Joe wrinkled his brow and invited Sam to help sort out how he could be helpful. Joe remarked that Sam didn't seem to need help planning his future. If anything, Sam could help Joe and the CFI business partners in this area. After 14 years, they didn't even have a business plan. Sam smiled when Joe acknowledged Sam's business-planning superiority, but his positive and confident demeanor also changed. He slumped in his chair, looked down toward the floor, and began mumbling about there being other problems—problems he had trouble talking about. This humble (nonhierarchical) conversational approach helped Sam to acknowledge what he knew and what he didn't know, and to identify where his confidence was high and where it was still low.

SAM: (*looking subdued and sad*) To tell the truth, the real problem with my future isn't with the business so much. I know I'll be able to handle that stuff. I know I can provide for my own family. I just don't know if I'll ever have a family.

ERON: Why not?

SAM: To have a family, you have to meet a woman, and I haven't done so great in that department.

ERON: Have you had woman friends?

SAM: Yeah. My last real girlfriend was in high school. I really liked her and trusted her, but I found out through the grapevine that she was sleeping with my best friend.

ERON: What did you do when you found out?

SAM: Nothing really. I just stopped seeing her or talking to her. I never confronted either of them. I didn't want to give them the satisfaction of seeing me upset.

ERON: Have there been other partners?

SAM: I've hung out with a few women since that time, but I'm afraid to get close to anybody. I just keep women at a distance.

ERON: I bet you must meet a lot of women through the store? You've got a lot of customers, don't you?

SAM: (*smiling*) No kidding. There's one regular customer that I'm really attracted to. Her name's Wendy. She's in the store a lot. I'm okay about finding batteries for her, but I break out into a cold sweat when I think of asking her out.

ERON: When I was single, I used to get into long rehearsals before the mirror, where I'd practice silly lines, then never deliver them. Do you do that one?

SAM: No. I don't even get that far. I just give up.

ERON: Sounds like that relationship in high school didn't help too much. How did things go before that?

SAM: There were a few girls that I saw, but I was always shy. I never had any confidence with dating. Now it's even worse. And forget it with sex.

ERON: What do you mean, forget it? I couldn't help but notice you light up when you started talking about your customer, Wendy. I was beginning to wonder why she drops by so often—how many batteries does a person need?

SAM: (*now looking sheepish and red-faced*) Since I found out about my girlfriend in high school, sex hasn't worked out so great. Sometimes I wonder if there's something wrong with me.

ERON: What makes you think something's wrong with you?

SAM: I don't last very long. And sometimes I think I might be gay.

TALKING ABOUT TRUST

Sam wanted to be seen as a trustworthy employer who was surrounded by reliable people, and he seemed more comfortable with people when he got to know them. He didn't want to follow in his father's footsteps as a cold and calculating businessman. He wanted warmer relationships with people. Since Sam preferred warmth and intimacy, Joe expressed curiosity about whether Sam had a different experience with women after he got to know them better. He inquired about the trusted others in Sam's life. Was there anyone in his past or present life whom he judged to be trustworthy and dependable? What happened in these relationships?

As Sam talked about trusted others in his life, he slowly regained his composure. He warmly referred to his brother and sister as people he could count on. He often confided in his older brother about his relationship woes. It was his brother who reassured him after his experience of betrayal with his high school girlfriend. Sam then described his unsuccessful experiences with women. He said that whenever he was truly interested in a woman he didn't know well or who didn't know him well, he either prematurely ejaculated or lost his erection during intercourse. Neither experience helped him feel very good about himself. Afterwards, he kept his discomfort and embarrassment about his sexual performance to himself and refrained from asking his partner about how she felt. Usually, an experience of sexual failure simply marked the end of the relationship. These disappointments added fuel to Sam's growing doubts about his sexuality.

When asked how he met women now, Sam said he enjoyed going to local dance clubs. However, if he danced with an attractive woman and she invited him to sit down and talk or have a drink, he'd move on briskly to the next dance partner. Later on, if he found his original dance partner attractive, he might go home and imagine what it would be like to get to know her more intimately, but he'd never go so far as to get her name and phone her. All this hemming and hawing and hesitation around women caused Sam to doubt his masculinity. Although he prided himself in being a take-charge, decisive man of action in the world of business, he saw himself as ineffectual around women. This contradiction disturbed him deeply.

SELECTING KEY STORIES

Sam wanted to see himself as a confident man who had a firm grip on a future that included marriage. Yet, his thought that women viewed him as unattractive and inadequate contributed to doubts about his sexuality and confusion about where he was heading in life. Sam's preference for open conversations and trusting relationships with others was unmistakable. Sam did not want to follow in his father's footsteps as business executive or intimate partner. He felt his father was insensitive to his mother's emotional needs and thought his mother too sensitive to his father's needs to speak up for herself. His parents did not have the kind of loving relationship he hoped to have with a trusted partner. (These views of self and other are summarized in the matrix of views in Figure 12.1.)

Taking into account this constellation of preferences and views, Joe asked Sam about his past experience with the women he truly got to know and trust. He was curious about whether Sam experienced different results when he engaged in more open (preferred) conversations with the women he found attractive. Sam responded by relating a key story about his 7-year relationship with Linda from Aus-

Vantage points	Sam
Preferred view of self	Confident, sensitive, attractive to women, capable of intimacy, different from my father.
View of significant others	My siblings are trustworthy. My ex-girlfriend betrayed me. **D.V.**—Women see me as inadequate, unattractive.
View of family of origin	My father was insensitive to people. My mother ignored her own emotional needs. My parents had a distant marriage.
View of therapist or other helpers	The therapist can help me gain confidence with women. He sees me as capable of intimacy.

FIGURE 12.1. Matrix of views.

tralia, a story that helped Joe understand the problem and find the solution.

LETTERS TO LINDA AND OTHER STORIES

Sam met Linda on her first visit to the United States, and they had carried on a correspondence ever since. Sam said he took more risks than he was accustomed to taking when he met Linda, because he figured she wouldn't be around long enough to hurt him. Other than his brother, Linda was the only person Sam confided in about his lack of sexual confidence. He told Linda about the betrayal by his high school girlfriend and how badly he felt about it. He told her about his perceived sexual failures and conveyed to her his worries about his inadequate performance. Linda was supportive, sympathetic, and reassuring. To his surprise, Sam had the rare experience of enjoying sex with Linda. He did not prematurely ejaculate or lose his erection. He felt comfortable with her and that she enjoyed their intimacy. He carried lasting memories of their time together. Despite a string of disappointments with other women, Sam continued to write letters to Linda, telling her of his frustration and hurt. And, in turn, Linda wrote to Sam about the trials and tribulations of her life and her relationships.

It was through these conversations about trusted others, and through this story of enduring intimacy in the wake of persistent failure, that the groundwork was laid for a narrative solution. Sam figured out that having *open conversations* was the key to building comfort and confidence in his sexuality. The next step was to link Sam's preference for open conversation with his desire to conduct relationships differently than his father, then to address the overarching question that marked Sam's entry into therapy, namely, Who am I and where am I heading in life?

The next bit of dialogue between therapist and client makes the connection between these key narrative elements, creating a coherent story line.

ERON: The story you told me about Linda helped me understand what you meant when you said you wanted to manage people differently than your father—with more sensitivity and concern. It's clear that when you use these instincts as your guide, you have good experiences with women. When you don't, things don't go so well.

SAM: I don't know what you mean exactly.

JOE: Remember when you were talking to me about how you intended to manage the family business? I noticed that there was no hesitation whatsoever in you about how to do things. You'd hire people you trusted. You'd get to know them as people and help them feel part of the operation. Basically, you'd make sure you did things differently than your father.

SAM: Right. Absolutely.

JOE: I noticed when things went well in your relationships with women, you followed the same principle. Even if the person you were attracted to was dazzling on the outside, you felt better when you got to know her on the inside, and when she got to know you on the inside. When that happened, it seemed that the relationship worked well. Sex worked well. You were comfortable, and she was comfortable. In other words, when you did things your way, things went well. When you acted more like your father—more distant and removed—things didn't go so well.

SAM: I guess I never thought of it that way. Maybe I do know what I'm doing more than I thought.

JOE: You're clear about the kinds of relationships you want to have. The only thing I don't get is where these doubts come in about your sexuality? You definitely seem attracted to women, and you know what it takes to have a close, comfortable relationship. You seemed pleased with your sexual performance when you had a relationship that fit your beliefs about how relationships should be. I'm puzzled about where this worry about sexual performance, or concern that you might be gay, comes from.

Although Sam had appeared empowered by Joe's comments about his clear sense of direction with love and work, he now looked dazed, his face turning pale and expressionless. Slowly, Sam gathered himself and said there was something he needed to talk about, but he hadn't quite drummed up the courage to bring it up.

"Please," Joe said, "don't feel pressured to talk about anything you're not comfortable talking about." But Sam insisted that he needed to get something off his chest. It was at this point that he began to speak about his secret.

SAM'S SECRET

Sam said he was 10 years old when it happened. There was an older teenage boy in the neighborhood who befriended the younger children. At first, Sam thought there was nothing out of the ordinary about an older boy wanting to be with younger boys, and he was proud to claim having an older friend. Then he started to realize that something was strange when the older boy made him do things he felt he wasn't supposed to do. He said he was instructed to perform oral sex on this boy and, somehow, strangely, experienced pleasure doing it. Sam remembered feeling frightened about putting up a protest, because the older boy threatened to hurt him if he told anybody—once brandishing a knife to support this threat. Sam never spoke with anyone about this abuse; however, he remembered that the reign of terror stopped after a neighborhood boy, who was also a victim of these acts, told his parents. He vaguely recalled that the boy's parents spoke to the perpetrator's parents, and the sexual abuse stopped. Sam never said anything about this disorienting and terrifying experience to an adult out of fear that his father would find out. Sam's father was drinking at the time. When he drank, he'd often go into hateful tirades about homosexuals. Sam figured that his dad would surely view him as homosexual if he knew about the incident.

Therapists know that these untold tales of sexual abuse can profoundly shape a person's life. It's not only the event itself that is upsetting and disorienting, but it's also how the event is storied. In Sam's case, the narration of this shameful experience went on privately. Sam's construction of this event shaped how he viewed himself in relation to other events in the normal flow of development, such as dating, high school dances, first sexual encounters, and early hurts and betrayals. Sam was never reassured by a parent, another important adult, or even a peer that he was okay. He was never told that a bad thing happened to him that was not of his choosing or initiative, and that he wasn't responsible for the results. Left to his own narrative devices, Sam came to compose a story of self that suggested he was defective, and not whole.

This negative story of self—shaped by the experience of sexual abuse and its silent influence, reinforced by his early disappointments with his high school girlfriend—affected Sam's experience with women as an adult. Although he wanted to be intimate with women, his experience of past shame interfered with acting in line with his preferences. When Sam concealed his wishes, needs, and insecurities from his partner, he experienced premature ejaculation or lost his erection. This experience of failure, in turn, corroborated the unsettling meaning of the untold story of sexual abuse, informing Sam that he was defective. This frame of deficiency was reinforced by the lingering experience of disjunction. Although Sam never spoke with his father, he imagined that his father would view him as gay if he heard Sam's story of sexual abuse. Because Sam vaguely recalled experiencing pleasure in the forced sexual encounter at age 10, he imagined that he harbored a secret preference to be intimate with a man. Given the history of his father's derogatory comments about homosexuals, Sam imagined that this secret preference was a sign of deficiency. Since Sam never spoke with his mother, sister, or brother about this event, he also felt that they would regard him as flawed if they ever heard his story. This case presents a vivid example of how stories affect frames and frames affect stories in the absence of intimate dialogue.

The evolving problem and the problem at its worst are portrayed diagrammatically (see Figures 12.2 and 12.3). It's clear from these diagrams that Sam's problem with confusion over his sexual identity is maintained currently by his withdrawn behavior around women, and his reluctance to engage in open conversations with them. Sam's story about his successful experience with Linda highlights the importance of intimate conversation as a solution to his sexual-performance difficulties.

Note that the revelation of Sam's secret followed a trail of helpful, nonintrusive conversations in which the therapist expressed interest in how Sam preferred to see himself. As Sam came to view the therapist viewing him as a competent man who took charge in ways different from his father, he grew more confident about speaking openly with the therapist about shameful things. He came to trust that if he shared his secret with Joe, Joe wouldn't view him as flawed or inadequate. By the time the therapist posed the mystery question to Sam about his shakiness about his sexuality (inviting him to explain why someone so clear about his preferences would act so uncertain about his sexual identity), Sam was confident enough to finally tell his story,

The Evolving Problem

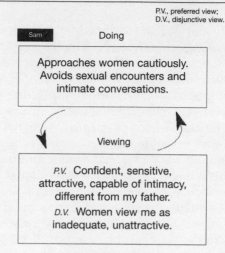

FIGURE 12.2.

The Problem at Its Worst

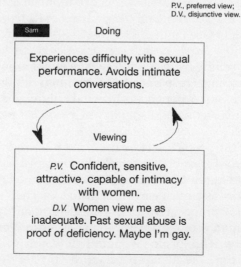

FIGURE 12.3.

filling in for the therapist the missing pieces of the puzzle of problem evolution.

THE RESTORYING OF SHAME

When Joe asked Sam if there were any current reminders of the sexual abuse, Sam mentioned that he'd had recurring nightmares since the age of 14. These nightmares further reinforced Sam's doubts about his sexual identity. He said their persistence had something to do with his decision to seek therapy in the first place. There were a few variations on the content of these dreams.

In one variation, Sam looked at himself in a mirror and saw his image change and become distorted. Sometimes, an unidentifiable man approached him from behind in a threatening way, then disappeared from view. Sam figured that this dream had something to do with the perpetrator of the sexual abuse, but he didn't know how to interpret its meaning. In another dream, Sam found himself looking at another man's body in a curious way. He wasn't sure whether this was a sexual dream, because he'd awaken in a cold sweat before any sexual encounter took place. Sam later volunteered that he found himself looking at men in real life as well. The purpose of these gazes seemed comparative, as Sam would measure himself against other men and find himself lacking. He'd never pursue the man he was looking at in a sexual or flirtatious way or have any desire to do so, but he'd nevertheless categorize his own urge to gaze as strange and somehow perverted.

Recently, Sam said, women were appearing more and more in his dreams. In one recurring dream, Sam was about to make love to a woman. When he moved toward her, a man appeared in the background and his attention was drawn to the man. This distraction interfered with the completion of what had been a pleasant encounter with his partner.

Joe talked with Sam about the meaning of his dreams. They discussed whether his real-life experiences (such as looking at other men) might reflect his strong preference to take charge of his future. Joe emphasized how Sam seemed the kind of person who wanted to look at himself squarely in the mirror and figure out who he was and where he was heading. Since Sam was interested in being a more introspective, sensitive man than his own father, wouldn't it be natural for him to compare himself to other men to gauge how he measured up? Sam seemed relieved about considering this alternative explanation. Joe remarked how it might be interesting for Sam to see how this curiosity would be expressed in the future as he gained self-confidence. With more confidence, would Sam look at other men, then look at himself and realize that he was okay? Or might he simply not need to make these comparisons so often?

Joe and Sam concluded that the recent content of Sam's dreams signified progress. That Sam now had dreams of looking at himself in the mirror while the threatening male figure disappeared into the background was a sign that he was beginning to separate himself from the terror of his past. That Sam was now imagining himself being intimate with women in his dreams was also a sign of his awakening self-confidence. He seemed ready to encounter women once again with newfound knowledge about himself.

These positive reconstructions of the meaning of Sam's dreams and real-life experiences weaved through the therapeutic conversation as Joe and Sam restoried the past and present and Sam's vision of the future. As Sam positively connoted the meaning of unsettling experiences throughout his life, he noticed his own strengths. (Note how the reconstruction of meaning in the therapeutic conversations reflects information in the matrix of views in Figure 12.1.)

GENERATIVE CONVERSATIONS OVER TIME

Sam became inspired to engage in new conversations. He now wanted to tell the story about what happened to him at age 10 with trusted others in his life. He chose first to talk with his sister, who was helpful to him. This successful conversation laid the groundwork for future conversations with partners-to-be. The next step, which turned out to be prophetic in shaping the future, was that he decided to write to Linda his most important letter yet.

In this letter, Sam retold the tale of sexual abuse at age 10, explaining as best he could how this event shaped his self-doubts. Linda responded with interest and compassion. Sam's disclosure drew Linda closer to him. She wanted to see Sam again and hoped to visit the States the following summer. As letters went back and forth to plan this future reunion, Sam made efforts to meet and date other women. Although he didn't meet anyone he felt interested in, the new conversations he had with women served to bolster his confidence. With one woman he dated a few times—someone he got to know and who confided in him—he actually summoned the courage to talk about his past experience of sexual abuse. Although the conversation went well, the relationship never developed into more than a friendship.

Slowly, Sam grew more confident about his sexuality and more hopeful about his future in love and work. As it turned out, Linda did visit Sam during the summer. They rekindled their romantic relationship, this time with more passion than before. Sam said sex was even better than the last time, because he felt Linda now *really* knew him, that he really knew her, and that their deeper knowledge of each other solidified their desire to be close. They parted with newfound excitement about their relationship and a commitment to write even more frequently.

Sam tried out a few more relationships during the next year, none of which fulfilled his requirements for intimacy. During that year, he negotiated the gradual takeover of his father's business, to be completed in 3 years. He said these business negotiations went well. He was comfortable once he decided to focus on discussing facts and figures with his father and avoiding emotions. (For a summary of the key ingredients of a narrative solution, see Figure 12.4.)

About a year after Sam's reunion with Linda, they arranged another get-together, this time in Australia. Sam got along well with Linda's family and said their commitment to each other grew even stronger. In the September following this visit, Sam wrote Linda and

A Narrative Solution

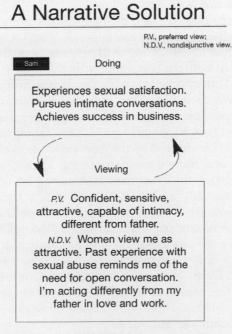

P.V., preferred view;
N.D.V., nondisjunctive view.

Sam   Doing

Experiences sexual satisfaction.
Pursues intimate conversations.
Achieves success in business.

Viewing

P.V. Confident, sensitive, attractive, capable of intimacy, different from father.
N.D.V. Women view me as attractive. Past experience with sexual abuse reminds me of the need for open conversation. I'm acting differently from my father in love and work.

FIGURE 12.4.

asked her to marry him. Ten days later, Sam received a letter back. Linda said she'd be willing to be Sam's partner in life.

About 2½ years and about 40 sessions after Sam's original statements of doubt about having a business and a family, he had both. Although Joe knew that Sam's story of the letters to Linda was a key in helping Sam be more aware of his preferences in intimate relationships, he never expected that highlighting this story would be a form of courtship leading to marriage. Today, Sam is the sole proprietor of a successful hardware business. He and Linda have a 3-year-old son whom they adore.

Sam stopped therapy after his engagement to Linda, but this wasn't the end of Joe's contact with him. The conversation continued intermittently over a period of 5 more years through a series of several important life transitions. Sam checked in with Joe soon after the wedding, and they met for four sessions. Sam reentered therapy after Linda became pregnant, and they met 10 times over a period of 3 months. Sam also came in with Linda after the baby was born to talk about the challenges of parenting and to discuss his fear of losing Linda to the baby. Recently, Sam and Linda came in for a few sessions to talk about their frustrations with the hardware business and their desire to get some distance from Sam's family. It has now been a year since Joe met with Sam or Linda.

What was the basis of these intermittent conversations? Were they helpful, or was Sam becoming too dependent on therapy and using it as a crutch? How does talking with clients in spurts, over a long stretch of time, fit with the concept of brief therapy?

Each time Sam checked in with Joe, it was around a key transitional event, and each time they returned to narrative themes discussed previously. For example, Sam became nervous during Linda's pregnancy about how he would turn out as a father, and how their relationship would be affected by the new baby. He noticed that he was spending more and more time glued to the TV and drinking beer. It was also during this time that Sam had one of his old sexually confused nightmares. Joe and Sam talked about how the daunting prospect of becoming a father naturally awakened concerns about who Sam was becoming as a man and father. This was an understandable time to have the old nightmares, to be sensitive to old habits that reminded him of how his father behaved as a father, and to take stock of what kind of father he wanted to become. Sam felt reassured and empowered by this explanatory frame. He cut down on his beer drinking and TV watching and started spending more time with Linda and the baby. The nightmares subsided.

Once Sam was reacquainted with his preferences and positive intentions, he stopped therapy for awhile. These intermittent conversations initiated at pivotal times of transition served as booster shots. Sam was immunized against old patterns of thought and action, and given an injection of confidence to move forward and manage the life transition at hand. Sam left each brief series of conversations with a stronger sense of what kind of man, husband, father, and hardware store owner he wanted to be.

One of the reasons that Sam continued to check in with Joe was that Joe became an important other in corroborating Sam's preferred identity. The untold story of sexual abuse had clinging power. It affected troublesome views of self and others over a long expanse of time. The therapist was the first person to hear and respond to this story, and in so doing, he confirmed how Sam wished to be seen. This placed the therapist in a privileged position as an important, trusted other in Sam's life. Naturally, Sam would want to talk with Joe when doubts were reawakened by an important life transition.

The delicate balancing act for the therapist is not to become too important. Conversations inside the therapy room need to strengthen conversations outside the therapy room. The therapist's job is to help people figure out how they wish to talk with intimate partners, friends, family members, bosses, and coworkers about such things as pregnancy, parenting, children, sex, closeness, television, beer, in-laws, and hardware stores. The idea is to generate helpful conversations with others that confirm people's preferences and positive intentions so that they become less reliant on the therapist as an intimate conversant. This intermittent-conversations approach becomes a way to respect the important position that the therapist assumes when hearing and interpreting untold tales that run people's lives (such as sexual abuse), without becoming so important that new conversations and new partnerships are blocked.

HOW BRIEF IS NARRATIVE THERAPY?

The case of Sam's secret raises the question: Is the narrative solutions approach brief therapy? In the last chapter, Tom met with a young woman who presented with a clear concern she called "OCD" and resolved the problem in five sessions. In this chapter, Joe worked with a young man who presented with the severe condition called "I'm not sure where I'm heading in life," and resolved the problem in 60 sessions over a period of 7 years.

Some possible explanations for this difference include the following: (1) Tom is a better therapist than Joe; (2) Tom is an expert on OCD, whereas Joe doesn't know much about sexual abuse; (3) Sam really had an underlying personality disorder that necessitated long-term treatment; or (4) Joe has a longer attention span than Tom.

Although all these explanations are plausible (in particular the fourth one), there are other considerations that may be more relevant. As we said at the beginning of this book, our experience has been that problem resolution (and the speed of problem resolution) has less to do with the types of problems people present, or the severity of their complaints, or the intrinsic qualities of individuals and families affected by the problem, and more to do with the nature of the talks we have with them. Still, it's interesting to speculate as to why some therapeutic conversations can be helpful in a relatively brief period of time, whereas other conversations need to go on over a longer span of time to be effective.

In the cases of Valerie and Sam, the therapists engaged individual adults in conversations about the mystery of problem evolution and learned that the problem had its social constructionist roots in childhood. Spurred on by Tom's questions, Valerie quickly identified how her OCD symptoms were originally linked to her upset over her parents' fighting at age 9. Valerie said that a previous counselor had clued her into this connection between symptoms and context. Valerie also said that her symptoms went away after her parents' fighting stopped and mentioned that they didn't reappear until recently. Thus, Tom was tapping into previous knowledge that Valerie already had about the evolution of her symptoms, and was reacquainting her with that knowledge. As Tom inquired further into the present symptom context, Valerie identified that once again she was being affected by the upsetting behavior of intimate others, in this case a boyfriend. As Tom and Valerie restoried the evolution of symptoms in both interactional contexts along preferred view lines, Valerie figured out what she needed to do in the present to get beyond her symptoms.

In Sam's case, Joe (in his slow, methodical manner) also engaged his client in a conversation about the mystery of problem evolution. Gradually, Sam identified how his current sexual confusion and anxiety symptoms were linked to the event of abuse that happened at age 10. This key event had been storied privately by Sam, and in the wake of subsequent relationship failures, a story of self as defective had prospered. In contrast to Valerie, whose symptoms were intermittent and not part of a fixed negative view of self, Sam's symptoms were so persistent that they affected his basic sense of identity as a person. Furthermore, Sam's symptoms and perceived identity were unaffected by new information about himself. Sam's sexual success in his intimate relationship with Linda hadn't altered his well-entrenched doubts about his sexuality or modified his defective view of self. This negative view of self didn't shift until the therapist drew attention to his positive experience with Linda, then punctuated how this successful experience was a consequence of Sam's acting in line with his own preference for open conversation and his wishes to be different from his father.

Once Sam acted in line with his preferred view by talking openly with the therapist about sexual abuse, this painful memory could be reconstructed in a self-confirming way for the first time. In this instance, restorying involved the introduction of new information about the self, and this new information needed time to assimilate before behavior patterns could change. Thus, the extent to which helpful solutions to problems can be brought about in a brief period of time seems a product of the resources, past and present, available to the therapist. The brief therapist remains on the lookout for resources inherent in people and their relationships with others that can be brought to bear on solutions. Therapists must also appreciate, however, that *they* are a relationship resource, and use this resource to promote helpful conversations with others inside and outside the treatment room. More important than how long therapy takes is whether therapy is helpful in breaking the patterns that bind people and empowering them to manage their lives effectively.

—13—

As Time Goes By: Conversations with Adults in Distress

E ven when it appears that we've completed the transition to adulthood, when we've "succeeded" at love and work, events happen, and we feel forced to start over again. The career we choose doesn't work out. The company relocates and we have to move. We decide to leave a relationship we're in and live alone; or, our spouse leaves and we're forced to be alone. We start dating, trying to form new partnerships, and become reacquainted with the awkwardness of feeling like a teenager again. We find a new companion and start a new family. We choose a mate who has her own children, and we try becoming a parent to these children.

The many changes and challenges of adulthood invite us to look back on the broad composition of our lives. Did we do what we set out to do? Did we act in line with our own preferences or bend to the expectations of others? Did we become who we wanted to be? Who can we still become? At midlife, we're inclined to pause, reflect, take account of our lives, and consider where we're heading.

At 38, Helen looked at her life and felt good about most of the choices she made. In keeping with her preferences, she lived her life differently from her parents and became the adult she hoped to become. But there was one thing she couldn't seem to change. It was a problem that had been around too long, and she was itching to resolve it.

RESTORYING HELEN'S HIVES

Helen came to therapy on the recommendation of her family physician. Her doctor treated her for several years, unsuccessfully, for chronic hives—a condition that dated back to her early teens. Over a period of 25 years, Helen tried a multitude of solutions. In her early teens, she relied on her mother's baths with baking soda and a range of medicines prescribed by different doctors. She tried homeopathic remedies, stress-reduction programs, hypnosis, meditation, massage, and women's groups. Although she found many of these approaches to be beneficial to her general health and well-being, nothing had really cleared up Helen's hives. There were times she was without hives, but these respites were few and infrequent.

Curiously, Helen was at a stage in her adult life in which she felt more "in control" and comfortable than even before. She had just completed a master's degree to advance her training as a critical care nurse and landed a well-paying administrative position at a local hospital. Three years prior to contacting Joe, Helen left a 7-year marriage to a man she now described as controlling and verbally abusive. She said that when she first met Jonathan, she was swept away by his charm, good looks, and luxurious life style. She was a country girl from humble roots, and he was a city boy from a wealthy and cultured background. They lived *his* life style, residing in a high-rise apartment on the Upper East Side of Manhattan. They went to fine restaurants, attended theater and ballet, and hosted elegant parties for elegant people. Helen felt that Jonathan introduced her to the finer things in life—things she hadn't known before but soon learned to enjoy. But, she also felt that he was in charge of what she said and did, that he ran their financial and social life, restricted her freedom of movement, and showed little interest in her ideas and emotions. During this marriage, Helen abandoned her nursing career to accommodate what she saw as Jonathan's preference for who she should be. She stayed at home to tend to the household and play host to their many guests, but she wasn't really happy with this role. Ultimately, Helen felt good about her decision to leave this relationship in which she felt she had submerged her voice and lost sight of who she wanted to be.

About a year after leaving this marriage, Helen met another man named Michael, who she said was very different from Jonathan. Like Helen, Michael was a helping professional and a helpful person. He worked in a residential treatment facility with adolescents—long hours with modest pay. He cared about his friends, about the troubled children he worked with, about his own family, about Helen's family, and most of all about Helen. Helen felt comfortable talking with

Michael, and Michael felt comfortable talking with Helen. He showed an interest in what she was thinking and feeling. She felt respected. Whereas Jonathan had discouraged contact with her family, sometimes finding fault with them for their uncultured ways, Michael showed a genuine interest in her three sisters, brother, and aging parents. When Helen's parents needed work done on their house, he'd offer his services. With Michael, Helen felt part of her family again and, in many ways, more herself.

The mystery question that oriented Joe and Helen's conversation was this: Why was a competent, independent woman who took such bold steps to reclaim herself—to locate her own voice, to rekindle and advance her career, to find a man who loved and valued her—still itchy and uncomfortable?

Helen was an introspective person, and she quickly responded to this question with a variety of interesting observations. First, Joe and Helen talked about the few exceptional occasions when the hives had either disappeared or diminished in intensity. Interestingly, one memorable 2-week period of remission came after the breakup from Jonathan, when she moved into her own apartment and was making plans to go back to college. Unfortunately, this brief reprieve from hives didn't last long. The turning point, she felt, was her brother's illness.

Helen's brother, Victor, was dying of AIDS, and she had become his sole confidant and caretaker. As his illness worsened, her sense of responsibility increased. During this time, the hives made a strong comeback. As Victor grew closer to death, Helen began to feel torn between her work, her brother, and her new relationship with Michael. Michael was supportive, often accompanying her on her visits with Victor, telling her that she should do whatever she needed to do, and that she needn't worry about spending time with her brother. But they were planning to marry in August, and it was Michael she wanted to be with. As Helen reviewed the evolution of her predicament, she realized that the hives went away for a brief time when she was *attending mainly to herself* and when her sense of responsibility for others was less pronounced. Helen was intrigued by this discovery but unsure what to do about it.

Looking Back

The theme of responsibility for others became the focus of the narrative search—both forward and backward. Helen began talking about how her responsibility to and for Victor fit in with her strongly developed orientation to care for others, which was groomed in childhood.

When Helen approached her teen years, she remembered wanting to make friends, wanting to take part in school activities, and wanting to go out with boys, but felt held back by family responsibilities. She recalled having to baby-sit for her younger sisters and help her father and mother around the house. She and Victor always had a close bond and talked with each other about their troubles, although she was more often the caretaker of Victor. Helen rarely voiced any discomfort about having any of these duties. She accepted her lot without protest but inwardly knew she was unhappy.

And what about the hives? When did they begin? Helen recalled that she was 14 when the hives first appeared. There was a boy she wanted to date, but her parents wouldn't let her. She put up a bit of a protest, but her words fell on deaf ears. The first bout with hives occurred during that time of protest, then compliance.

And what about her experience with dating after that time? Helen recalled that she submerged her normal teenage desires from that point on. Her youth was filled with responsibility for others, she said, and it wasn't until her college years that she explored relationships with men for the first time. Looking back, she realized that her inexperience and lack of confidence had a lot to do with her fascination with Jonathan. He was experienced and worldly. Her vision was that he'd take care of her and teach her to be a confident woman. No wonder her hives went away after leaving Jonathan. Helen could see that this was the first occasion since expressing a preference to her parents to date at age 14 in which she spoke up about her own wants and needs. And she did it with a man she once put on a pedestal and allowed to assume a parental position in her life.

Joe's interest in Helen's views of other family members also turned up important clues to a narrative solution to hives. For example, when Helen described her mother, she said that she, too, suffered with chronic hives.

"How was your mother when it came to taking care of herself?" Joe asked.

"Are you kidding!" Helen said. "My mother's never done anything for herself in her life. My father depends on her for everything, and it's gotten worse in recent years since he retired and became ill. My mother can't ask for help from anyone else in a direct way. I'll give you a perfect example. The other day I was at the house, and she asked if I was going to the supermarket later. I told her I wasn't planning to. Then she said something like, 'Oh, come on. There must be something you need to pick up at the store, isn't there?' I said, 'No, not really, what do you have in mind, Mom?' 'Oh, nothing,' she said. 'I guess I was just hoping that if you were going, you could pick up some aspirin. Never mind.' Then I asked if she was having trouble with her headaches again, and she said not to worry. That's my mother—she can't ask for anything. I went to the store and brought her back the aspirin, and she seemed to be annoyed with me for putting myself out. You can't win."

Joe inquired as to whether Helen hoped to follow or not follow in her mother's footsteps. She said she was clear that she wanted a life different from her mother. That's why she was so attracted to Jonathan. She thought he could take her away from her restrictive family life and make her a new person. But she realized that linking up with Jonathan was a mistake. Although the accoutrements of life in her first marriage bore little resemblance to those her mother had, she had acted a lot like her mother in her relationship with Jonathan. It was no wonder her hives persisted in this marriage and cleared up when she decided to leave it. But what was going on now? Why did the hives make a comeback?

This discussion of past events helped Helen pinpoint how hives fit into her life. She clarified her preference to be different from her mother, to be more self-oriented and speak up about her needs. Now it was time to apply this new knowledge about the early evolution of hives to her current situation.

Looking Forward

Joe asked Helen whether she talked about her own needs with her brother Victor. Had she sought *Victor's* help in figuring out how to balance competing preferences—the wish to be with him alongside her strong desire to be with her husband-to-be? Helen clarified that she hadn't talked about herself with Victor at all. She focused only on him and his compelling needs. Then Joe remarked, "Didn't you say that you and Victor were close while you were growing up, and that he was the one you talked with when you were upset?" Helen agreed that this was true. Joe then said he was puzzled: "Why wouldn't you talk about yourself with Victor? Wouldn't he benefit as well from such a talk? Wouldn't talking with Victor about yourself *help him* in some way to feel part of your future at this final short period in his life?"

Helen seemed moved by this way of looking at things and decided to talk with Victor in a new way. She and Joe then explored whether it made sense to talk with Michael about her feelings of overresponsibility. Although Michael had always encouraged Helen to spend as much time with her brother as she saw fit, she now realized that this wasn't the kind of support she needed. What she really needed was to talk with Michael about their wedding.

Helen also decided to engage Michael's help in figuring out how to spend less time with her brother yet still feel like she was a good sister. Joe had helped Helen notice that she was following in the footsteps of her own mother by not asking for help in a direct way. She was doing her own variation on the aspirin story. This was a prohive approach and Helen wanted to take action to reverse it.

New Conversations, New Solutions

Helen took charge of her present situation by talking with her brother, Victor, and her husband-to-be, Michael, about her preferences. She spoke with Victor about her wish to be there for him during his illness and plan her wedding with Michael. She also talked to Victor about some of the things she and Joe talked about—growing up together, their parents and siblings, Helen's first marriage, her newfound confidence, her desire to be true to herself, and her excitement about starting a new family with Michael. Helen felt Victor was pleased with this conversation, and he expressed his hope to be there for her wedding. He encouraged his sister to spend time with Michael and acknowledged that it might be a good idea for him to spend more time with other members of the family, rather than with just Helen. Helen felt enormously relieved by these conversations and even closer to her brother. She started to feel comforted herself by visiting with him, in addition to being of comfort to Victor.

Helen also talked with Michael about her wish to attend to their wedding plans and her conflict about focusing on her brother and neglecting herself. Michael supported Helen's efforts to talk about herself with her brother and bring other family members into the helping network. He suggested that Helen talk with her sisters about their wishes and concerns, and she did. This conversation with her sisters went well. They expressed an interest in spending more time with Victor and also encouraged Helen to plan her wedding. Further conversations ensued with friends and family about how to make the wedding a special event.

It was in the wake of these new conversations that Helen's hives disappeared. They stayed away even during the intense time of her brother's death which, sadly, occurred just before the wedding.

After 15 sessions, Helen's symptoms dissolved. She and Joe have had intermittent conversations since that time about new events in her life, such as the birth of her first child. At one point, the hives made a brief comeback when she decided to move back into her parents' home to take care of her father when he was severely ill—this at a time when she was pregnant and hoped to focus on her new family. After one session with Joe, Helen realized that she was getting back into a prohive pattern. She decided to have a helpful conversation with her parents and husband about what to do differently. After Helen moved out of her parent's home and decorated a room she and Michael added for the baby, the hives went away again. They haven't returned. Helen has been free of hives for 2 years now, and she seems clear about how to conduct her life in the future so that they stay away. Should her hives return, she now knows what to do to alleviate them.

Adults may wind up in our offices even when they've formed meaningful partnerships, completed successful careers, raised children and steered them into adulthood; then they watch their children start careers, find meaningful partnerships, and have their own children. Even when the life cycle has flowed with a gentle merry-go-round rhythm, harsh things can happen to break the flow. Retirement doesn't go as expected. Illness or infirmity strikes.

ILLNESS AND DISJUNCTION: A CASE OF DEPRESSION IN AN OLDER MAN

The next case is of a 65-year-old man named Al who had recently retired. About 2 years after his retirement, which was going along reasonably well, he was diagnosed as having chronic emphysema by a trusted family physician. In subsequent meetings with his doctor about his physical symptoms, Al revealed that he was feeling depressed, withdrawn, and "not his old self." He was referred by his physician for treatment of depression brought on by his illness.

When Joe greeted Al in the waiting room before their first meeting, he noticed first his large, powerful hands. They enveloped Joe's as if to suggest that Al was the one who was supposed to be helping Joe feel more secure in this relationship. Soon, Joe learned that Al prided himself in being someone who could work with his hands. He viewed himself as a real family man, the main breadwinner, and prime caretaker of a large family that consisted of his wife, eight grown children, and 15 grandchildren. Everyone came to Al when they had a problem, when something needed repair, or when someone needed financial advice or assistance. Al's retirement didn't change his position in the family. There was still always something to do, something to fix, someone who needed his help or advice.

But the emphysema really threw Al for a loop. He felt that he was no longer the person he used to be. Now he sat around all day feeling depressed and useless. What was worse, he said, was that he felt distant from his family and that they noticed it. When Joe asked Al to help him understand what his family noticed, he told a story that captured his current predicament.

The Snowfall: A Key Story about Problem Evolution

After a recent snowfall, Al went out to shovel the driveway, an old and familiar job for him. He went at it full tilt, as always. But 5 minutes into the task, he started having difficulty breathing and became quickly frustrated. In disgust, he threw his shovel in the snow, retreated to the house, and collapsed on the couch, where he spent most of the day. His wife and son came around to talk to him, but he didn't have much to say. When Joe asked what happened to the driveway, he said that later, without saying a word to him, his son went out and finished the job. A pained look came over Al's face, as if this were a final blow, proof that he was no longer the man he used to be.

Having heard this story, Joe asked Al to help him understand what he envisioned for the future when he watched his son finish the snow-shoveling job from his withdrawn perch on the couch. Al remarked that he pictured himself turning out to be just like his own father. "What would that be like?" Joe asked. Al said that his father became a different person after he retired from his job. Like Al, his father had been an active, productive, helpful, center-of-the-family person until the time he retired. Soon afterward, he turned inward and became reclusive and unproductive. Only 2 years after his retirement, Al's father died suddenly of a heart attack. Al pictured himself following his father's example. However, he didn't want to be remembered by his children in the last years of his life as he remembered his own father. This idea of the future deeply disturbed him.

Joe then asked Al how he thought his wife and grown children were viewing him now. Did they notice changes in him, similar to the changes he had noticed in his own father after his retirement? Al said that his family regarded him as different, as "not his old self." No one had asked for his help with anything in some time, and everyone seemed to keep their distance from him. "How did that feel?" Joe wondered. "Was it more comfortable to feel removed from your wife and children, or did it feel better to be an active part of their lives?" Al said that it was terrible to feel so separate from his family—that was the worst thing that had resulted from his recent depression.

At this stage in the conversation, we had enough information to diagram the evolving problem cycle from Al's point of view (see Figure 13.1). As you can see from this diagram, the onset of emphysema had seriously shaken Al's preferred view of self. He had always wanted to see himself as a hardworking, productive family man but now,

The Evolving Problem

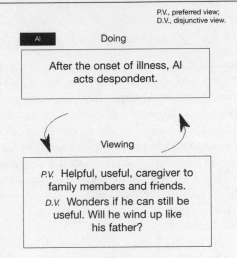

P.V., preferred view;
D.V., disjunctive view.

Al   Doing

After the onset of illness, Al
acts despondent.

Viewing

P.V. Helpful, useful, caregiver to
family members and friends.
D.V. Wonders if he can still be
useful. Will he wind up like
his father?

FIGURE 13.1.

along with his breathing, this preferred view had come under strain.
His self-doubts were aggravated by the idea that he might wind up
like his father, who soon after retirement became an inactive recluse,
then suddenly died.

Recalling Preferred Stories

Having mapped the evolving problem cycle from Al's point of view,
Joe then inquired about what life was like in the family before the illness and before he became depressed. What were things like when Al
felt more active, useful, and involved with his family? Al described a
life filled with acts of helpfulness and close family involvement. One
key story that emerged from this inquiry involved Al's profoundly retarded daughter, who lived with the family until the age of 25. He said
that one of the most difficult decisions that he and his wife ever had to
make was to place their daughter in a residential facility. They realized
that they couldn't provide the care she needed anymore, and they supported each other through this difficult period of separation. Ultimately, the decision worked out well for everyone involved. The reason
that this was a key story was that it highlighted an important issue relevant to the successful management of Al's illness. This past story
showed how Al had once been capable of *recognizing limits* and knew

how to initiate a helpful conversation with his wife to support these limits.

After hearing the story about Al's daughter, Joe asked Al whether there were other occasions in the past when limits needed to be set and he took charge of the situation. Al responded by talking about his problem with drinking many years before. At one point, when Al got word from his family physician that drinking was affecting his health, he decided to stop. He did this on his own without seeking professional help. When Al announced his sober intentions to his family, they were pleased and supported his efforts at self-control. Thus, Al revealed himself to be a disciplined and determined person who could set realistic limits, who could make important and difficult decisions, and who could direct others about how he wanted them to be supportive. These stories from the past offered clues to the solution. They revealed strengths and positive resources that could be used to change the present situation. Having elicited these key stories of mastery, success in setting limits, and directing the support of others, the therapist posed a mystery question. How was it that a man who had managed so many difficult things in his life, who had known how to set realistic limits and take charge of his family, would find himself in a position where he no longer felt in charge? This question peaked Al's curiosity. Joe suggested that he meet with some members of his family to pursue how they actually viewed the current situation, and to see if they too could be helpful in unraveling this mystery. Al supported this idea.

After only one session with Al's wife and two of his sons, it became clear that they were floundering. Al's illness, they said, had turned their beloved father and husband into someone they didn't know. They had no idea what to make of his illness, no facts, no direction, no sense of what Al could still do, what they should do, and so on. What Al regarded as loved ones viewing him as useless had actually grown out of their own sense of helplessness. Family members preferred to view themselves as caring and helpful. When they saw Al acting despondent and withdrawn, they tried to lift his spirits by encouraging him to cheer up. When this didn't work, they became even more confused about what to do.

Family members viewed Al viewing them as unhelpful, which propelled more of the same solicitous behavior. As they began completing tasks for Al, such as shoveling the driveway, Al became more convinced that the people he cared about viewed him as helpless, and he grew even more depressed.

The more despondent and withdrawn Al acted, the more solicitous family members became, and the more delicately they approached him. A diagram of the problem at its worst can be drawn,

The Problem at Its Worst

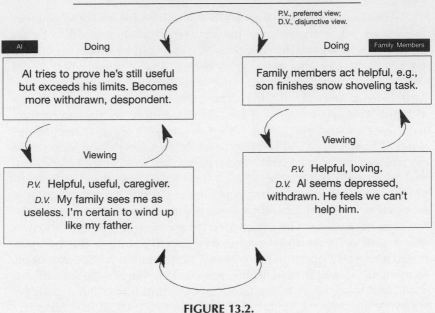

FIGURE 13.2.

which now includes the views and actions of family members (see Figure 13.2).[1]

In the next session with Al, Joe used verbatim quotes from his conversation with family members to emphasize their bewilderment. Joe mentioned that they were "floundering" and had no clue about what Al was capable of doing. Joe described how family members actually viewed Al since his retirement, noting how pleased they were with his positive adjustment to this transition and how active he had remained. He also mentioned what Al's wife said about her memories of her father-in-law. She, too, recalled his rapid deterioration after re-

[1]The reader may wish to return to Chapter 2 and compare the assessment of this problem to the MRI approach to a similar case. You can see once again that in the MRI approach, attention is focused on the behaviors that maintain problems and on persuading people to reverse problem-maintaining behavior by following therapeutic directives. In this case, attention is drawn to the *views* of self and other that propel the problem into motion and keep it going, as well as the *actions* linked to these views. Furthermore, in this case the therapeutic conversation is conducted with the person suffering the illness, and family members are brought in to assist in the process. In the MRI case, only the stroke victim's family participated in therapy, not the stroke victim himself.

tirement but felt strongly that Al was *not* his father and *would not* follow his example. Al's pattern of behavior following retirement convinced her that he would stay active and connected with family members, unlike his father. Joe also shared with Al the sadness that family members expressed about his recent emotional withdrawal—how they didn't seem to know quite how to approach him, or how to ask for his help anymore, and how much they wanted him back in the family again. Joe said that family members were wallowing in confusion at a time when they most needed Al's guidance.

Al Takes Charge

This conversation with Al about the intentions, preferences, and needs of his family helped to alter the disjunctive attributions that emerged in the wake of retirement and illness. Al began to view family members as preferring to have him be his old self and regarding him as still capable and helpful to them. This reconstruction of current events, supported by preferred recollections from the past, inspired swift action toward a solution. Al immediately came up with the idea that it was high time to sit down with his doctor and find out what he could and could not do. He entered this meeting from an empowered position, equipped with detailed questions. After finding out that he could still do many things, but at a more moderate pace, he sat his family down and explained the facts of his illness to them. When Al started to approach tasks at a more comfortable pace and complete them, his despondency lifted. He later mentioned that he joined a self-help group for emphysema sufferers, and, true to his old form, assumed a leadership role. He even seemed to be breathing easier.

The problem resolved when Al began to see others seeing him in ways more compatible with his preferred view (see Figure 13.3). As he took charge of his illness and acted more like his old self, family members backed off and resumed interacting with him in familiar ways. Family members began to see Al seeing them in ways that promoted their own preferences. They now knew better how to be helpful and felt more confident that they could once again ask Al for help without upsetting him or aggravating his illness. Now that they could count on Al to counsel them about his limits, their sense of burden lessened.

TO RECAPITULATE

The subjects of the two case stories used in this chapter, Helen and Al, illustrate how the past can be a resource in working with adults to pro-

A Narrative Solution

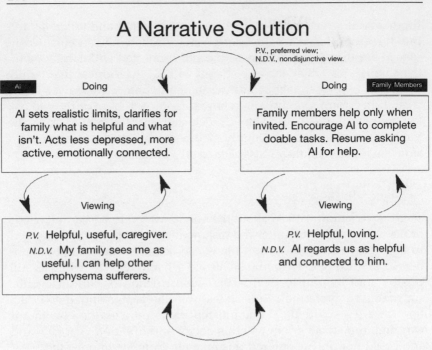

FIGURE 13.3.

mote rapid problem resolution. In Helen's case, the origins of chronic hives were traced to Helen's teenage years, when she first tried to assert her independence and met with parental disapproval. Helen followed in her mother's footsteps, although she never wanted to. Helen's mother also suffered with hives and had difficulty "living in her own skin," as Helen poetically put it. Helen attempted to chart her own independent course into adulthood but couldn't quite shake the hives. The therapist helped Helen recall past exceptions to the occurrence of hives. Helen related that she was free of hives for a brief period after leaving her first marriage. The hives made a comeback when she became preoccupied with her brother's illness and once again submerged her own wants and preferences. Once Helen became clear about the origins of hives and figured out how these symptoms fit into the fabric of her life, she quickly figured out what to do to relieve her symptoms.

Al became depressed after developing emphysema but had a long history of life without depression. This extended history was used by the therapist to reacquaint Al with his preferences and restore in his mind who he once was and still is in the eyes of others. Al soon realized that he *could* set realistic limits, and that his family still needed him. Al altered the worrisome idea that he was following in the path of his father, who deteriorated after retirement and the onset of illness. Al changed his image of the future. Al's depression quickly resolved as he reconstructed *present* symptoms in the context of *past* life experiences.

Brief therapy can incorporate the breadth of the life cycle and still be brief. The narrative solutions approach allows therapists to identify strengths and resources over an expanse of time. Therapists needn't restrict their focus to here-and-now problems and solutions in order to achieve rapid change. Brief therapists can help people develop a cohesive storyline that explains how current problems fit into the tapestry of their lives. Not only do clients leave therapy with symptoms improved or eliminated, but they also depart with a blueprint for how to manage life's future challenges.

—14—

When Things Get Complicated, Part I: A Collaborative Solution

T hus far, we've discussed the application of our approach to a variety of problems that crop up at different stages in life. For purposes of clarity, we've not discussed cases with complex entanglements—when family members are embroiled in conflict, when clients are mandated for therapy, or when problems demand the involvement of multiple agencies. For the most part, we've described talking with people who wanted to talk with us.

How do you talk with people who don't want to talk to a therapist—who are only in your office because they feel forced to be there by others? How do you proceed when people are in extreme conflict with each other, yet they refuse to talk with each other, except through their attorneys? What do you say (if anything) to attorneys when you feel that legal action being pursued by family members only perpetuates their conflict? How do you engage family members who are adamantly opposed to therapy and appear zealously committed to the legal battling, yet you feel that their participation in therapy is essential to finding a solution? The following case addresses many of these complications.

SALLY'S STORY

Three years before our contact, 9-year-old Sally's parents divorced. Based on her parents' mutual decision, Sally went to live with her father, Peter. One year after the divorce, Sally was diagnosed, then treated for leukemia. When Sally's mother, Jane, called to make an appointment for Sally, her leukemia was in remission. Sally was living with Jane temporarily and, as we learned, her parents were in the early stages of a court battle over custody.

Here's the initial telephone conversation with Jane:

LUND: I got your call and wanted to speak with you briefly.

JANE: I'd like an appointment for my daughter, Sally. I'm really worried about her. She's often crying. She refuses to go to school . . . I'm concerned she might hurt herself.

LUND: Has she indicated that she might?

JANE: The reason I finally called was because I found her sitting in the bathroom late last night (*tears*) with a coat hanger around her neck. She was crying and saying she wanted to die.

LUND: Did it seem like she was really going to hurt herself?

JANE: I don't think so. It was just hanging loose, and she said she had been sitting there for awhile. I think she was asking for help. I want her to be seen right away.

LUND: Sure. Have you or other family members ever done this before?

JANE: Yes, I saw Dr. Eron at your place about a year ago, and I saw other therapists before that.

LUND: Was it helpful?

JANE: Yes, I think each therapist was helpful in a different way.

LUND: Was anyone else interested in your making an appointment for Sally?

JANE: People at Sally's school are concerned because she's missing school so much, but I'm doing this on my own.

LUND: Are other family members interested in participating?

JANE: That doesn't matter to me. It helped me, and I would like Sally to express her feelings and work them through.

LUND: So family members are for it.

JANE: Well, her father isn't. He's dead set against therapy. He was when we were married and always will be. He will not participate, I'm sure. But, this is for Sally. I wish Peter would, though. He could use it.

LUND: What's his view of therapy?

JANE: He thinks people should be able to solve their own problems. You wouldn't like what he says about therapy.

LUND: But I'm interested.

JANE: He thinks it's whining, finding excuses, and avoiding doing something about your problems.

LUND: You seem to know a lot about his ideas of therapy.

JANE: He told me often enough when we were married, and I was in therapy. I think he blamed one of my therapists for the breakup of the marriage.

LUND: So he doesn't live with you folks?

JANE: That's a long story.

LUND: In that case, let's make an appointment and we can talk more.

JANE: Sally isn't too sure about this. She says she doesn't want to talk with anyone but me about her feelings. I'm not sure she'll meet with you alone.

LUND: That's okay. We can all meet together.

JANE: That sounds good . . . actually I would like you to meet with her alone so she'll tell you how she feels, not influenced by me.

LUND: Let's see how it goes when you get to the office. If Sally will talk with me alone, we'll do that.

JANE: You should also know I have contacted an attorney to help.

LUND: How is the attorney helping?

JANE: I think I'm going to sue for custody.

LUND: Oh, that's a good thing for me to know.

Just 9 months before this telephone conversation, shortly after Jane stopped therapy with Joe, the family had a party to celebrate Sally's remission from leukemia. The party was planned by Sally's mother and father. The entire family attended, and everyone had a great time. According to Jane, Sally didn't experience any serious emotional problems during the entire period of her leukemia treatments. Now, in remission, Sally was found with a coat hanger around her neck and was refusing to go to school.

When Jane and Sally arrived at the office, Jane gently encouraged Sally to talk with Tom alone. Sally followed her lead with little resistance.

Sally entered the therapy room wearing a brown wool cap that covered her closely cropped hair, still thin from chemotherapy. This sad-eyed, frail 9-year-old looked down at the floor and spoke softly as she responded to the therapist's questions. Tom began by letting Sally know the little he knew about why she was there.

LUND: (*in a soft voice*) You know I talked to your mom the other day, and she told me a little bit about what's going on lately. I don't know much. I like to meet with folks your age first to understand how you see things, rather than talk too much with the adults.

Sally nodded. Her eyes briefly lifted from the floor and met Tom's, then returned to their original place. But she said nothing.

LUND: Your mom said something about your being at her house, but that you used to live at Dad's?

SALLY: (*eyes still fixed on the ground and speaking almost inaudibly*) Mom and Dad are divorced, and I'm at my mom's apartment.

LUND: Oh. Where is that?

SALLY: On Berne Road.

LUND: So you go to the Mills School. What grade?

SALLY: Third. But I'm not there much lately.

LUND: Your mom said something about that . . . you haven't felt too good.

SALLY: My stomach hurts.

LUND: Is Mom helping you with that?

SALLY: She tries. She took me to the doctor, and she talks to me a lot.

LUND: You talk a lot about something helpful?

SALLY: Kind of . . . we cry together sometimes.

LUND: Cry together . . . why are you crying?

SALLY: I cry because I miss Mom. She cries because she has no one to cry with.

LUND: How come she has nobody to cry with?

SALLY: She lives alone. My brother and I live with my dad.

LUND: I think I'm confused. I thought you lived with your mom.

SALLY: I'm there now, but I live at my dad's.

LUND: How did that come to be?

SALLY: I missed my mom and called her from camp. Dad got mad. He said I should stay at camp, but Mom came and got me. Dad got pretty mad. I stayed at Mom's after a while.

LUND: Oh, so you stay at Mom's now and visit Dad?

SALLY: No, I don't visit Dad (*tears welling up*). He's mad.

LUND: This doesn't sound so good.

SALLY: It isn't so good.

LUND: How do you know Dad is mad?

SALLY: (*long pause*) I called him on his birthday from Mom's and he said, "You've hurt me more than you'll ever know."

LUND: He said that?

SALLY: Yes. (*tears*)

LUND: But you wanted to call Dad and were thinking of Dad on his birthday.

SALLY: I do think of Dad, but he's mad.

At this point, Sally spoke at length about how her father, his new wife, and her siblings all lived in a big house, while her mother lived all alone in a small apartment. She spoke of a dream about her mother being eaten by a spider and not coming to pick her up at summer camp. This spider dream occurred just before Sally's desperate call to her mother to retrieve her from camp.

LUND: You certainly are a thoughtful girl. Calling Dad on his birthday, even when you knew he might be mad at you. Is Dad mad at anyone else?

SALLY: Mom.

LUND: They don't seem to be getting along right now?

SALLY: No, the police even came over.

LUND: The police?

SALLY: Mom brought me to Dad's to pick up some stuff, and I was playing with my dog. Mom got mad. She thought Dad wouldn't let me go. She started kicking the door, then she called the police.

LUND: How was that for you?

SALLY: It was bad. Mom was upset.

LUND: What happened?

SALLY: I stayed with Dad.

LUND: Was that okay?

SALLY: Not for Mom. She called. Dad wouldn't let her talk to me. He said I was all right.

LUND: When was this, when you were staying with Mom or Dad?

SALLY: It was in the summer after Mom got me at camp.

LUND: You stayed at her house for awhile, and that was how you got back to Dad's?

SALLY: Yes.

After a short while Sally got weary of talking. Tom then asked Sally what she liked to do. When she said she loved to draw, he asked if she would draw him a picture. Sally asked what Tom would like her to draw. He couldn't resist asking her to draw a picture of herself. The picture said a lot about how Sally felt about herself and her situation. A girl in tears, frowning, with arms positioned stiffly by her side, was crossed out. It seemed that Sally didn't want to project this negative image of herself and suddenly changed her mind and drew a different picture, a more preferred portrait. Although not smiling, this little girl's mouth appeared to be inching in the direction of a smile. Her hair was stylish, her arms opened wide, and she appeared freer from upset.

After talking with Sally, Tom walked her back to the waiting room and invited Jane to speak with him. Jane was a tall, attractive woman, dressed in warm colors; she greeted Tom with a cheery smile and a firm handshake.

LUND: Sally was very open and articulate. She gave me a clear picture of herself and how she feels.

JANE: (*raising her eyebrows and looking a bit surprised*) That's good. I was worried she'd feel like I dragged her in here. I thought maybe she wouldn't talk to you. She only seems to want to talk with me.

LUND: Well, she certainly spoke up. We could have gone on for a long time.

Tom intentionally highlighted Sally's comfort in talking with him. This set the stage for Jane to think of herself as a competent mother who made a sound decision about bringing Sally for therapy. Tom steered the conversation toward Jane's previous success in helping Sally go to school.

LUND: This business of doing what's best for Sally in spite of her resistance isn't new.

JANE: No.

LUND: You do a bit of that to get her to school.

JANE: Sometimes it works, sometimes it doesn't.

LUND: When does it work?

JANE: I'm not sure. I think when I feel strong and she doesn't feel stronger. She has been forced to do things that she hasn't liked for her own good before.

As Jane recalled helping Sally do things she was fearful about, the conversation naturally turned to the ordeal of the leukemia treatments. This key story revealed strength and determination on the part of all family members. It also demonstrated teamwork between the parents and the people-strengthening power of that teamwork. Gradually, Jane filled in her story of the evolution of the problem—and described the curious way in which collaboration turned to conflict for this family.

JANE'S STORY

Four years before the recent crisis began, Jane and her husband, Peter, divorced. At that time, Sally was 6 and her older brother, Jason, was 9. Feeling confined by an "emotionless" marriage, Jane sought to find herself. She went back to school, developed a new circle of friends, and tried to reclaim a vanishing sense of independence. Because her children said they wanted to stay with their father, Jane saw this as the best temporary arrangement. She moved to an apartment and visited with the children every weekend.

Jane described Peter as a stiff, stoic fellow, not one to show his emotions. The separation proceeded like the marriage, without outward displays of emotion or anger. Jane portrayed Peter as handling the breakup with grim determination. After a few months, he abruptly announced that he wanted custody of the children. Although shaken by the suddenness of Peter's decision, Jane acquiesced to save the children from an ugly court battle. A mere 3 months after Jane granted custody to Peter, and with little time to even assimilate the permanency of this new arrangement, the awful news came. Sally was diagnosed with leukemia.

Over the next 3 years, what the parents did was incredible. They worked together, sharing the responsibilities of transporting Sally to and from the hospital, supporting her through the treatments and painful tests to evaluate whether the treatments were working. Jane and Sally usually took the long ride together in the car, chatting and consoling each other. As they talked, Jane encouraged Sally to express her inner emotions and responded to Sally's fears and tears with warm reassurance. Peter often met them at the hospital. Jane said she couldn't bear seeing Sally in pain, so Peter took on the grim job of helping Sally get through the extremely painful tests. Sometimes Peter literally had to hold her down for the physicians to do their unenviable job. Jane described Peter as intolerant of any outward displays of emotion on Sally's part.

During the time of the treatments, Peter remarried. Shortly thereafter, Jane contacted Joe to be seen individually. She was feeling guilty about some of her past decisions, and was concerned about how Peter's new wife, Janice, might affect their teamwork.

After only a few sessions, Jane reported feeling stronger. It was she who invited Peter and Janice to a therapy session so that they could all confirm their continued commitment to work together for Sally. They all joined in optimism about the prospects for remission and discussed plans for a future celebration. After therapy ended, Jane continued to date and make new friends, completed college, and launched what would soon turn into a successful career. When the good news finally came, the family celebration went off as planned.

Jane recounted this portion of the narrative with obvious sadness, but she spoke in matter-of-fact terms. Her steadfast optimism found its way through the cloud of despair that now surrounded her. It was not until she spoke about the present situation that the warm, cheery smile witnessed in the waiting room completely evaporated into tears. Somehow, Sally's remission created an opening for all the sadness about the marriage, the loss of her children, the ordeal of Sally's illness, and the pain of past mistakes, to come pouring out.

As Jane talked, it became clear that she wished to see herself as a caring, attentive mother who was willing to make sacrifices for her children. This commitment had its roots in her early experience with her own mother, who was alcoholic. Jane felt that her mother was never there for her emotionally. She vowed to herself early on that she would always be tuned in to her children's emotional needs. She explained to Tom that it was this commitment to spare her children inner turmoil that motivated her decision to grant custody to Peter and avoid a custody battle.

THE EVOLVING PROBLEM

During the summer, Sally complained to Jane about how badly she was being treated by her older brother, Jason, and stepbrother, Gary.

After weeks of hearing complaints, Jane approached Peter on Sally's behalf. She didn't get the response she wanted. She felt that Peter was insensitive to Sally's emotional needs. He made it clear that he and his new wife, Janice, were determined to get things back to normal in their home. They felt that Sally was spoiled by the adults due to her illness, and it was time for the other children to get some of the attention they deserved. Peter and Janice expected Sally to pitch in and manage routine responsibilities of the household like everyone else. When Sally put up a fuss, Peter and Janice scolded her. Then the boys got on Sally's case, and Sally called her mother, who called her father, who wasn't too sympathetic.

Sally's complaints and Peter's gruff, let's-get-back-to-normal attitude prompted Jane to rethink her decision to grant Peter custody. She remembered Peter's insensitivity in their marriage and now felt that Sally had taken her former place as the victim of this insensitivity. When Sally was receiving the painful treatments, Peter's stoic approach was an asset. Now his approach seemed cruel. Jane worried about how Sally would manage in this unemotional household where children were expected simply to do what they were told.

During the summer months, after the news of remission, Sally went to Girl Scout camp. She called her mother every day to tell her how much she missed her. One day, she described a nightmare in which her mother was eaten by a spider. Having been swallowed by the spider, Mom wasn't available to pick Sally up from camp and return her home. Hearing this story, Jane immediately rushed to the camp and brought Sally back to her apartment. She informed Peter about the incident later. He was beside himself with rage. According to Peter, Jane had spoiled Sally once again, give in to her fears, and didn't even consult him about her impetuous decision.

The school year brought with it more complaints from Sally about missing her mother. Then came the stomachaches and refusals to attend school. These stomachaches were greeted by Peter with indifference, by Jane with worry and intense conversation. Jane began keeping Sally home from school on the days she was with her. She also began keeping Sally longer than the agreed upon visits. At first, Peter fought against these violations of their agreement, then he began to capitulate. At one point, he declared, "The two of you deserve each other."

On one occasion, Jane wanted to keep Sally for a few extra days, and Peter acquiesced. Jane brought Sally to her father's house to pick up the clothes she needed for her extended stay. Sally remained in the house. Jane called to Peter to send Sally out, but he didn't respond. (As Peter later told the story, he was watching Sally as she contentedly played with the dog and talked with her brother. Since she seemed to have no interest in going with her mother, he did nothing.) In reaction to this seeming indifference, Jane proceeded to kick the door. When there was no response, she called the police. When the police finally arrived, they said that since the father had custody, Sally should stay with him.

At this point, things really heated up. The family's normal routine could be easily disrupted by a hysterical phone call or cry for help. One day Sally called her mother from her father's house before anyone was awake. Crying uncontrollably, she insisted that she couldn't possibly go to school and needed to be with her mother. Jane advised Sally to wait until her father woke up, then call her, and she'd come over.

As Jane told the story, when Peter realized that Sally called her mother without his permission, he became livid. He laced into Sally for being sneaky and manipulative, and stormed off to work in a huff. When Jane arrived, Peter was nowhere to be found. Jane simply asked Sally what she wanted to do—to go to school or to her mom's house. Not surprisingly, Sally chose to go with her mother. Jane took the day off from work and stayed with her.

At this point, Jane kept Sally at her house, against Peter's objections. Jane would get Sally to school on some days and not on others. Soon, chaos and uncertainty ruled the family. No one was in charge of where Sally should live, who should care for her, or what should be done about her problems.

In the second conversation with Sally, Tom followed up on a portion of Jane's narrative about the evolving problem.

> "Sally, I just wanted to thank you for being so open and helping me understand what things are like for your family. I should have mentioned this before, but when I chatted with your mom, she let on that you're a very strong girl. That's why I guess I'm not as surprised as I'd usually be to learn so much from someone your age. She said that you'd been through some pretty rough stuff with leukemia, but that you got the best of it."

Looking pleased, Sally told Tom the details about the long needles and painful treatments. Like her mother, she told this story in a matter-of-fact way, without tears or obvious sadness. She described how her father would refuse to let her cry and sometimes held her down to get through the treatments. She seemed proud about how brave she was to get through this ordeal. She talked, too, about the long car rides with her mother to the hospital, and how Mom always made her feel better with words of comfort. The image she gave was of parents who acted like a team, even though they really had little to say to each other. Somehow, Sally's illness had brought out the best in both parents, allowing their individual strengths to flourish. Jane's warmth combined with Peter's toughness offered a healing blend.

Astonishingly, the ordeal of leukemia didn't produce a problem. Conflict between Sally's parents emerged only after Sally's illness went into remission, and this conflict seemed the basis of Sally's distress.

This assessment of problem evolution brings us to the next step. According to Jane, Peter was dead set against therapy and refused to participate. He and Jane were not presently on speaking terms and both hired attorneys. Tom could guess from Jane and Sally's descriptions that Peter preferred to be seen as a take-charge man who could weather adversity. It seemed he regarded Sally as spoiled and needing to toughen up in order to weather the challenges that were still ahead of her.

SETTING THE STAGE FOR SOLUTIONS

After assimilating Sally's and Jane's stories, two things crucial to achieving a successful outcome became clear to Tom. First, because of the extreme adversarial situation that now existed, Tom couldn't afford to wait long before engaging Peter in therapy. There remained missing pieces to the mystery of Sally's symptoms that only Peter could fill in. There was also a danger in developing a negative view of Peter based on others' stories. Peter was beginning to sound like an insensitive, uncaring person, and the therapist didn't want to join in seeing Peter that way, at least, not before meeting him.

The second and related issue was that a court battle didn't fit with the goals of therapy. Conflict between the parents was the basis of the evolving problem. Bringing the parents back together to work in Sally's best interests seemed the basis of the solution. Collaboration wasn't likely to happen within the adversarial constraints of legal battling.

These two issues, Peter's participation and the court battle, were addressed at the end of the second session with Jane.

LUND: I'm still amazed at how you and Peter put your differences aside when Sally needed you to rally around her in her fight against leukemia. Then you became unsure as to whether Peter appreciated Sally's emotional needs and whether he'd work with you in that arena.

JANE: He sees Sally as a spoiled brat . . . almost as if now that she's better, she should be paid back for having gotten so much attention . . . she should just be tough and ignore all of the feelings she has about leukemia and her parents' divorce.

LUND: He seems to be putting her feelings, her emotional needs aside.

JANE: He did that with me.

LUND: You seem to be able to keep Sally's emotional needs paramount. You avoided a court battle to protect Sally.

JANE: Yes.

LUND: At this point, you're going to go to court?

JANE: I'm not sure. I don't want to, but Peter won't even talk to me.

LUND: I wonder if we could engage him here?

JANE: I really doubt it. I'm telling you, he really doesn't like therapists. Besides, my lawyer said not to have contact with him . . . that we should speak only through our lawyers.

LUND: But if you could work together with Peter once again, you would like to avoid court?

JANE: Definitely.

LUND: Sometimes I talk with attorneys so that they know who I am and how I work with children.

JANE: If you and he could figure out how to talk to Peter, that would be good.

LUND: Do you think he knows that you would rather not go to court?

JANE: I told my lawyer that I would much rather negotiate this than go to court.

LUND: Even if Sally stays with Peter?

JANE: (*pause*) Yes, I think so.

LUND: You really want to do what's best for Sally. It's still not as important to you who Sally lives with as it is to really know what's best for her and to do it.

JANE: Of course I want her to live with me. I do think that's best. But I'm not doing this so that she lives with me. Does that make sense?

LUND: It makes a lot of sense for Sally.

Note that the negotiations around talking with Jane's attorney and inviting Peter to participate in therapy flowed out of a conversation about Jane's preferences and intentions. The therapist connected with Jane as a competent, caring mother who was willing to take an independent stand when her daughter's emotional well-being was at stake. He didn't challenge Jane's perceptions about Peter's insensitivity. Instead, he emphasized Jane's interest in doing what was best for Sally and his own interest in talking with attorneys about matters that affect children.

A CRUCIAL CONVERSATION WITH AN ATTORNEY

After this second session, Tom contacted Jane's attorney. The conversation went as follows:

LUND: Mr. Schwartz, my name is Dr. Tom Lund. I'm a child psychologist in town. I've seen Jane Friedman's daughter, Sally, on two occasions and wanted to talk with you about her.

MR. SCHWARTZ: I think we met once in family court. I've not met Sally yet. I'm glad she is seeing you. She's been through a lot in her life.

LUND:Yes. Her mother and I were speaking about that and how important it is for her parents to get along around her.

MR. SCHWARTZ: I guess Jane has been trying to get along. She seems to have given in and given in to this guy for years. She seems to be standing up now. He doesn't seem interested in cooperating.

LUND: Jane and I spoke about getting Dad in here.

MR. SCHWARTZ: I don't think that will go anywhere. Isn't he against that? Look, I don't think Jane can stand up against him. I don't like the idea of her talking with him.

LUND:You know, funny things go on when I speak with parents about their views of their children and their caring for them. Also, I'd be surprised if Peter's attorney would advise him to take a strong stand against having his daughter see a psychologist, with all she has been through. I'm not sure he'd look real good in court. I wouldn't meet with them together.

MR. SCHWARTZ: Actually, I don't see how trying to get him in your office could hurt. It might even help, if he refuses. Like you said, if he refuses, he won't look good.

LUND: If Jane agrees, how about if I call him and at least get the lay of the land? Then you and I can speak again.

MR. SCHWARTZ: That sounds good, as long as you don't set up a meeting with them together.

At this point, Tom called Jane to let her know the results of his conversation with Mr. Schwartz. Tom said he preferred to contact Peter himself and invite him to meet with him individually. He said that he wanted to gauge whether Peter would be interested in learning more about Sally's emotional needs. After all, that was really what Jane was interested in, more than a court battle. Jane eagerly agreed.

ENGAGING A RELUCTANT PARENT

By going with Jane's preference to meet with Sally for the first appointment, rather than pushing to engage all family members immediately, important clues were gathered about how to converse with reluctant participants. Before telephoning Peter, the therapist, with Jane's and Sally's help, already had assembled a picture of who Peter preferred to be. He assumed that Peter wished to be seen as an authoritative father whose intentions were to do what was best for his daughter, and to help her toughen up, to weather adversity.

However, certain contradictions stood out. For example, this take-charge father was putting his daughter's life in the hands of the legal system. He was also taking a backseat while his ex-wife, with whom he disagreed, took charge of his daughter's emotional well-being. He was acting as if his own point of view didn't count. The therapist felt prepared to speak with Peter and to engage his cooperation by addressing these contradictions.

The telephone conversation went as follows:

LUND: My name is Tom Lund. I'm a child psychologist. I don't know if you know that I've met with your daughter Sally. Whenever I see young children, I want to be sure to talk with both parents.

PETER: (*gruffly*) What can I do for you?

LUND: Well. I know that you're the custodial parent, the parent who took charge of your daughter after you and Sally's mother separated.

PETER: Yeah, yeah. That's correct.

LUND: I've seen Sally now on *two* occasions and I'm not comfortable about going any further without your involvement.

PETER: Well, you know . . . (*hesitating*). To tell you the truth, no offense, but I'm not so hot on therapy. This seems to be Jane's solution to all the world's problems. She's always going from this therapist to the next, and I think it creates more problems than it solves. Now she's dragging Sally to a therapist, and I can't say I'm too happy about it.

LUND: Well, I hate to say this, but I'm getting the impression that therapy's going to be the order of the day here. I know from experience that if things go along as they seem to be . . . with lawyers and family court . . . there'll be mental health evaluations and therapists along the way. In fact, courts often tell families whom they should see. Families usually don't have much choice in the matter.

PETER: I suppose that's what we've got in store.

LUND: I just felt I should tell you . . . I don't like to form opinions about kids without meeting with both of their parents, particularly without talking to custodial parents. It seems like things went pretty well when you were in charge.

PETER: Well, I'll think about it. I'm concerned that with this therapy, Sally's going to think she has emotional problems when she's just fine. She just needs to go to school and do the things that are expected of her, and have her mother stop spoiling her.

LUND: I'm not going to be able to help Sally without you. It's clear from Sally that she needs her dad. Think about it, and give me a call. I'll put off seeing Sally again until I hear from you. By the way, I should tell you that Jane asked me to call her attorney. She agreed to suspend the custody dispute if we can all figure out what's best for Sally.

PETER: Listen, I'll talk to my attorney. I'll get back to you about it.

The telephone conversation with Peter was crucial to the outcome of this case. The therapist attempted throughout to connect with Peter's preference to be an authoritative parent who wasn't inclined to defer authority to others. He framed participation in the adversarial legal process as an act of deference, predicting that mental health professionals and other evaluators would be imposed upon Peter. He offered Peter the alternative of working with him (a professional who viewed him as he preferred) or working with someone selected by the court. The therapist refrained from advising Peter about what to do. Instead, he commented on how he preferred to be helpful to children and parents under these strained circumstances.

In a week, Peter called back to make an appointment. By that time, Tom had spoken with Jane's attorney, who, in turn, spoke with Peter's attorney. Both lawyers encouraged the parents to try to settle the matter through counseling, without going to court.

PETER AND JANICE'S STORY

The session with Peter and his new wife, Janice, filled in many of the missing pieces of the puzzle about how the family's problem evolved. The therapist mentioned how struck he was with Sally's openness in discussing her ordeal, with her fortitude and determination in handling the leukemia treatments, with her dependence on her father to stay tough and get through them, and with her reliance on her parents' teamwork throughout the process. Peter agreed with and embellished Tom's statements. Tom then posed a mystery question to Peter and Janice: How was it that a young girl with these obvious strengths and survival skills, surrounded by such determined and caring parents, wound up in such a troublesome fix—missing school and talking about dying?

The story Peter told underscored his positive intentions. He felt concerned that after all the attention Sally received from family, teachers, and friends during her illness, she needed to toughen up and get back to normal as soon as possible. He and his wife, Janice, made a special effort to place the same expectations for household responsibilities on Sally that were there for the other children. This change in policy may have inspired Sally's complaints to her mother about the unfair treatment she was getting at her father's house. Peter attributed much of the blame for Sally's present condition to Jane for giving in to Sally's fears. He also expressed hurt about Sally's persistent phone calls to her mother. He regarded the phone calls as a rejection of his authority. But as he talked, it became clear that this seemingly insensitive and uncaring man was deeply troubled about his daughter and feeling powerless about how to help her. This sense of powerlessness explained his recent capitulation and desperate participation in a court battle.

Janice shared Peter's view that Sally needed to be treated like a normal 9-year-old. She, too, felt that Jane contributed to Sally's upset, but her strongest view was that both parents needed to calm down. It became clear that Janice's views and actions did not contribute significantly to the evolving problem. If anything, she would encourage Peter and Jane to resume working together in Sally's best interest.

By the end of the first session with Peter and Janice, Peter seemed more comfortable with the idea of therapy. He saw the therapist seeing him as a caring father who'd helped his daughter through tough situations before and as needing to be there for her in the future. He was reminded of who he was as a person, recalling his important role during the leukemia treatments and remembering how he took charge as a father after the marital breakup.

Most importantly, he resonated to the feedback about how Sally saw him, which included verbatim quotes from the therapist–child conversation. He softened as he heard about how much Sally relied on him. At the end of the session, Peter mentioned that his own anger and upset weren't helping the situation. Janice took his hand, looking pleased.

THRICE-TOLD TALES (FROM STORIES TO VIEWS)

After we heard Sally and her parents' stories of the evolving problem, we were able to complete the matrix of views, providing a summary of the key views of self and others that shaped the present predicament (see Figure 14.1). Scanning down the matrix, it's easy to see how disjunctive views developed for each person. Jane, Peter, and Sally all came to see an expanding cast of others seeing them in ways that were distasteful. These gaps in perspective accounted for the emotional intensity and the narrow range of views and actions that sustained their crisis. Tom began the task of highlighting people's preferences and intentions in a way that narrowed these troublesome gaps.

In his next individual session with Jane, Tom followed up on what he learned from Peter and Janice. He mentioned that Peter and Janice were active participants in the conversation, especially Peter. Tom recounted how they discussed Sally's leukemia treatments, recalling how brave she was and how well everyone worked together. Tom described Peter's concerns that things get back to normal for Sally, that she take on more age-appropriate responsibility at their home. Jane appeared to understand why Peter might be motivated to put the painful leukemia treatments behind him and return to "normal" life. She allowed that he was probably under pressure from Sally's brother and stepbrother to stop giving so much attention to Sally. Tom emphasized how Peter acknowledged that his own anger and upset weren't helping Sally get back to normal family life.

Jane seemed pleased to hear that Peter showed a measure of sensitivity to Sally's plight and took responsibility for his own actions. Thus, Jane began to reconsider Peter's intentions in a way that confirmed how she herself wished to be regarded. She appeared open to

Vantage points	Jane	Peter	Sally
Preferred view of self	A caring mother who will make sacrifices to meet her children's emotional needs.	A take-charge, caring father who is the main source of Sally's strength and discipline.	Caring about all family members.
View of significant others	Sally needs more emotional support than her father can give her. **D.V.**—Sally sees me as not there for her emotionally. Peter is insensitive to Sally's emotional needs. **D.V.**—Peter views me as "spoiling" Sally. **D.V.**—Friends question whether giving up custody was in children's best interest.	Sally needs to develop more strength and determination. **D.V.**—Sally sees me as insensitive. Jane is too soft, "spoils" Sally. **D.V.**—Jane sees me as insensitive and a bad father. **D.V.**—My other children see me favoring Sally.	
View of family of origin	My mother was unavailable to me emotionally.	My father was a take-charge, caring man who I looked up to. **D.V.**—My father questions my competence.	My mother sees me as a loving, caring daughter. **D.V.**—My father sees me as "spoiled" and uncaring. He is angry and hurt.
View of therapist or other helpers	Therapy is helpful.	Therapy is not necessary or helpful.	Following Mom's lead about therapy.

FIGURE 14.1.

considering an alternate explanation for the current predicament that was less negative and rigid.

RETELLING SALLY'S STORY WITH PETER

Following this session with Jane, Tom met with Peter alone. Tom again recalled Sally's positive comments about Peter's role during the leukemia treatments and his leadership during and after the divorce.

He said that Sally seemed puzzled and distressed that her father, who had always been calm, reassuring, and in command (even holding her down during the leukemia treatments as she fought him), had left it to her to decide whether she wanted to have a relationship with him. Peter reeled, seeming upset at first, but then admitted that throwing up his hands and telling Sally and Jane that they "deserved each other" was probably a big mistake. He announced that he wanted to get back in control but felt Jane was getting in his way. Tom steered the conversation back to Sally's point of view about both parents. He said:

> "Sally seems worried about her mother and whether she's okay. Sally has always looked to you as the strength, the person who refused to get upset and let negative emotions like fear and anger run the family. Now she feels she has the power to upset *even you*, when you never flinched in response to her fears about the leukemia treatments. She now worries that you might not be able to handle her emotional needs as you did her physical needs. This department has been turned over to her and her mother, whom she already worries about."

The therapist's comments implied several mystery questions, namely: Why would a strong, loving parent who always rallied to care for his daughter defer control to his ex-wife and daughter when they were already overwhelmed with worry? Why would he join in all the emotion and upset? Why would he participate in a court battle with Jane, placing the family's future in the hands of strangers, when his daughter was at a point where she was threatening her own life?

Peter looked pensive. He also appeared on the verge of tears, but was holding himself back, perhaps just as he held Sally back when he felt her emotions were taking over during the leukemia treatments. Peter then announced his intention to talk with Sally. He wanted to tell her he loved her, to reassure her that he and Jane would work things out.

Peter then asked Tom where he thought things were going in terms of the custody dispute. Tom said that he'd call Peter after talking with Jane.

RETELLING SALLY'S STORY WITH JANE

In the following session, the fourth with Jane, Tom and Jane discussed Sally's emotional needs and moved further toward a solution.

LUND: I wanted to lay out what seem to be Sally's concerns so that we can address them together. First, Sally was worried that she was not being treated fairly at her father's, that people started being mean, that Dad started expecting Sally to be "normal" from his point of view. This all seemed to convince her that he was no longer supportive.

JANE: Basically, she seemed worried that he didn't care, that she didn't deserve any attention . . . that Jason and Gary were being favored.

LUND: Second, Sally began to worry that her father was angry and perhaps didn't love her.

JANE: I think that's true.

LUND: So Sally is seeing you as supportive, as helping her with these worries, but then starts worrying that you are not okay, that you might not be there for her.

JANE: I'm not sure that's true.

LUND: What?

JANE: That she worries if I am okay.

LUND: I guess I interpreted the dream that the spider ate you to mean that she worried you could not protect yourself, that you might not be there for her.

JANE: Yes, I might not pick her up. That's really why I felt I had to pick her up at camp, but not that I'm not okay.

LUND: That's true. You know and I know that you're fine, but when you're worried that your father isn't there for you, you probably wonder if Mom will be there, and if she will be okay. Sally told me that she cried with you, and you helped her with her worries, and you cried with her because you were alone. She also mentioned that she lives with Dad in a big house, and that you live alone in a small apartment.

JANE: Do you think I'm making her worried?

LUND: I think that you are there for your daughter and would do anything for her, and I certainly don't think your daughter has anything to worry about regarding her mother.

JANE: But I have talked about my sadness about Sally not being with me.

LUND: Sally has been getting pretty worried since things escalated. The last worry, is it the fourth?

JANE: Yes.

LUND: Sally seems worried that her parents, who worked together and put their differences aside to support her leukemia, giving her strength and determination to face a life-threatening illness, are at war over her now. Her distress is at a point where she considers ending her life. Sometimes I've wondered if Sally, in her young mind, might even think that being near death might get her parents cooperating again.

JANE: I don't want to be at war.

LUND: You've made a huge sacrifice to avoid involving the children in a custody battle already.

JANE: I know what I have to do.

LUND: What do you have to do?

JANE: I have to return Sally to Peter's home.

LUND: Why do you say that?

JANE: I would love to have Sally with me, but I don't want Sally to worry about me. I always told her I was happy the way things were. I can't put her and her brother through a custody battle. She already worries that her father and I cannot get along. We have to. How would my getting custody help Jason, how would it help Sally's worry that her father doesn't care? He would be even more angry.

Although Jane seemed to be moving toward a solution, Tom was concerned that this decision resembled a previous decision in which she allowed Peter custody after their marital separation, a decision she came to reconsider after Sally's remission.

LUND: What about your concern about Peter meeting Sally's emotional needs?

JANE: He would have to agree to come to counseling for as long as you thought it was needed . . . until Sally felt supported by him . . . until there was less jealousy between the children.

LUND: This sounds like an incredibly difficult decision.

JANE: (*through tears*) It is. You have no idea.

LUND: You'll do whatever it takes to help your daughter.

JANE: I hope that I always will.

FROM DIVISIVE CONFLICT TO COLLABORATIVE SOLUTIONS

As we discussed the contingency that Peter would have to meet Sally's emotional needs, Jane elaborated on her list of demands about what needed to be managed in counseling. Shortly after this session, Jane had a very interesting conversation with Sally, strikingly different from the tearful exchanges that had become their ritual. She called Tom and said she told Sally that she loved her and felt that it was best that she be with her dad, who also loved her. She reassured Sally that "she would be just fine" and Mommy would "work with Daddy" to make sure Sally was happy. She then returned Sally to Peter. She explained to Peter that she would not seek custody as long as Sally, Jane, and Peter worked with Tom, and until both parents were satisfied that things were going well for Sally. Peter agreed to these terms.

After a few days at her father's house, Sally tried out the old routine. She called her mother before her father awoke, complaining of stomachaches and demanding that she stay home from school. Jane responded by telling Sally not to worry, that she'd be right over to the house. To the therapist's amazement, Jane recounted how she and Peter sat Sally down, reassured her that she had to go to school, and informed her that Mommy and Daddy would decide what was best for her. Peter and Jane then drove Sally to school together. On subsequent days, Peter insisted that Sally go to school and, with Jane's support, encouraged her *not* to call her mother. After about 2 weeks of assuming this collaborative approach, Sally's stomach upset and school refusal stopped.

Therapy continued for a total of 15 sessions during which time Sally did discuss her feelings about the separation and the illness. Most importantly, both parents talked to her about these events, indicating to Sally, in effect, that they were now codirectors of the "emotional department." Peter sought advice about how to handle Sally's continuing need for attention, much to Jane's pleasant surprise, and Jane stopped engaging in tearful conversations with Sally, much to Peter's pleasant surprise.

There have been three follow-ups with this family since therapy ended. Two years after the final session, Peter called to request our records so that Sally could enroll in a new school. Six years later, Jane called to discuss some adolescent issues Sally had mentioned, along with concerns about the most recent family transition of Jason going off to college. Finally, there was the "old meeting in the aisle of the supermarket follow-up." When Tom ran into Jane 2 years ago at his favorite place, the Grand Union, Jane reported that Sally was doing just fine in college.

The problem resolved as the gap narrowed between how people preferred to be seen and how they imagined others regarded them. Jane began to notice her strengths as a parent and saw Sally seeing her as a caring mother. Peter began to notice his strengths as a parent and saw Sally seeing him as a competent father. Peter and Jane even began to acknowledge positive attributes in each other. Mutual blame and negativity diminished. Sally noticed changes in both her parents. She saw them let go of the court battle and once again function as a unit. She saw both parents seeing her as a caring daughter who was sensitive to the needs of family members, and as a strong, determined girl who could weather adversity.

With these changes in perspective came dramatic changes in action. The parents united and "took charge." They took charge in a way that fit within a new story about how Sally's problem evolved and what she needed. The parents did not drag Sally off to school. Nor did the therapist participate in a tug-of-war with the parents to get them to take charge. The parents' teamwork combined elements of reassurance and firmness that resulted in Sally's regaining confidence about going to school. The parents collaborated with other adults, including school authorities and attorneys, so that Sally saw all of them working together, but with her parents clearly positioned as captains of the team. In this sense, structural changes and adjustments did take place but without pushing against the existing structure directly or assuming that there was anything really wrong with the structure in the first place.

Beyond just handling the school avoidance problem, Sally's parents began rebuilding her confidence to tackle the problems that lay ahead in life. As the family confronted new transitions and challenges that bred doubts and fears, Jane and Peter knew what to do. Their teamwork remained intact.

CONCLUSIONS

This case illustrates how to promote collaboration when families are immersed in intense conflict, and outside agencies become involved. Collaboration often requires hard work, perseverance, and initiative on the part of therapists. Teamwork isn't achieved by cheerleading for people to work together as a team, or necessarily by mediating heated disputes between opposing parties in the room.

In the narrative solutions approach, collaboration is promoted by therapists arranging and generating a series of helpful conversations between people interacting around the problem, and focusing their attention on concerns shared in common by all. In this case, the common concern was Sally. Sally's mother, father, stepmother, relatives, and teachers all wanted to act in Sally's best interests, even though their own conflict temporarily detoured them. As it turned out, even the parents' attorneys, engaged to represent their individual interests, co-operated in suspending the custody dispute to do what fit for Sally. The therapist inspired collaborative solutions by engaging the people involved in the conflict in a sequence of individual and conjoint conversations aimed at figuring out what was best for Sally.

Helpful conversations with important others outside the family (in this case, attorneys), who exert influence over problems, follow the same principles as for family members. We try to understand people's preferences and appeal to their intentions, whatever their positions of influence. We proceed with a plan by arranging conversations with reluctant participants after first consulting the people most motivated to define problems and seek help. In this case, the clues for talking with a reluctant father came from talking with a concerned mother and a distressed daughter. The therapist took charge, by himself initiating a crucial conversation with the mother's attorney, once he realized that the attorney's cooperation was essential to problem resolution. The conversation with Jane's attorney wasn't initiated, however, until Jane's cooperation was invited. In fact, Jane guided the therapist's "strategy" of conversation by clarifying her own preferences and intentions. The therapist's success in speaking with Jane's attorney, in turn, sparked a helpful conversation between the attorneys. These talks allowed the therapist to work with both parents and paved the way for them to reclaim control over their lives and families.

Being the center of everyone's common interest, Sally, too, contributed to a collaborative solution. Sally's story highlighted the urgency of adult cooperation and focused attention on what she needed to reclaim her resilience. When all was said and done, parental leadership was restored. Attorneys backed off, a stepparent and siblings cooperated, and Sally returned to her old self.

—15—

When Things Get Complicated, Part II: Mandated Therapeutic Conversations

When people act irresponsibly they often become involved with social agencies, such as child welfare agencies, probation departments, drinking and driving programs, and courts. People caught drinking and driving can lose their licenses. Parents who are alleged to have abused their children may have their children removed from the home. On occasion, social agency staff recommend evaluation and/or treatment by mental health professionals as part of their mandate.

People who come to us because they are required to usually aren't too happy about it. They may have a "problem" that we readily see, that others close to them see, that social agencies see, but somehow they don't see. From the mandated client's point of view, the problem may be the intrusive actions of the social agencies or the inappropriate concern of certain family members. When working with mandated clients, it's important to recognize and appreciate the impositional context of the therapeutic conversation.

Using a case example, let's describe some of the special considerations to keep in mind when working with people who are forced to see us. Let's also consider what to say to the people whose job it is to ensure that clients follow up with treatment and maintain prosocial behavior.

HOW TO TALK WITH A MANDATED CLIENT

John ("Butch") was 19 years old when he first called for an evaluation mandated by his probation officer. His mother, Marge, had tried to coax her son to get professional help on previous occasions, but he always refused—and she always backed off. She had been worried about his drinking since he turned 14. This time, she didn't need to push, because Butch got himself into trouble with the law. He was driving around with friends and, after being cut off by another driver, decided to make his outrage known. He leaped out of his car in a rage and threatened the other driver with a hammer, which he waved menacingly for all to see. A fight ensued, and a bystander called the police. This wasn't Butch's first scrape with the law, but this was the first time he was placed under arrest—and it scared him. Butch was mandated by the probation officer for alcohol evaluation as part of a presentence investigation (PSI). The probation officer hoped that this might lead to counseling for Butch.

At CFI, we have staff who specialize in treating specific problems. Butch was the kind of person that our partner, Timothy Adams, CSW, often succeeded in helping. Tim has a 20-year background in the treatment of substance abuse and knows how to talk with young people who behave irresponsibly. He also understands how to talk with parents, probation officers, law guardians, lawyers, judges, school officials, and others in the often large cast of helpers who become engaged in conversations with youth who get into trouble.

Often, when we're asked to take on a case that seems impossible—when people are acting out of control, imbibing dangerous substances, scaring and intimidating other people, or talking in inscrutable ways—we ask Tim if he's interested. He usually is. When others are blinded by the obnoxious or bizarre nature of a person's outward appearance or behavior, we trust that Tim will find a way to connect with positive qualities that others may not see.

As an example, Joe recalled two occasions in which people approached him at social gatherings and said, "You work with Tim Adams, don't you? Say hi to him when you see him, okay?" Later, when Joe got to the office and passed on these messages to Tim, Tim recalled that these were people whom he had evaluated on charges of driving while intoxicated (DWI). In New York State, DWI offenders are forced to receive evaluations by experts in alcohol and substance abuse, who then make specific recommendations to the State Department of Motor Vehicles about whether their licenses should be renewed or revoked, and what kind of treatment services, if any, should be provided. Both men who approached Joe were people Tim recommended should *not* drive under any circumstances, and should instead become involved in intensive treatment programs. Usually, people who are recipients of such news aren't too happy with the messenger, yet these men wanted Joe to "Say hi to Tim!" Although this seemed curious, we assumed that Tim found a way to conduct conversations with these men such that a well-concealed preference to be more in control, to be viewed by others as responsible, or even to be monitored closely by others, came to the fore. Thus, a recommendation to relinquish a license and engage in treatment became a natural outgrowth of a conversation about preferred views. Somehow, the recommendation became the client's as much as Tim's.

After Tim's first few meetings with Butch and his parents, Joe asked him how things went. He said that this case was a "piece of cake." "Sweet kid, nice parents, everyone seems motivated. I talked with the probation officer, and even she's enthusiastic about family therapy."

Tim thought this was an easy case. He had positive resources within the family to work with, a 19-year-old who wasn't too put out about having to come for therapy, and helping agencies that wished to be cooperative with treatment. Yet, he was also talking with a young man who was arrested for threatening a stranger with a hammer, and whose mother and stepfather felt had been out of control with his drinking since the age of 14. As it turned out, Tim met with Butch and his parents in different combinations for 10 sessions over a period of about 6 months. During that time, Butch made a decision to stop drinking, reapplied and was accepted to college, began conversing with his immediate family in new ways, maintained sobriety with friends at social gatherings at which others were inebriated, stopped acting violently, and renewed contact with his biological father for the first time in 8 years. Tim's response to these results was, "Butch and his parents were ready to change. I happened to come along at a good time."

Although we knew there was probably some truth to what Tim was saying, we also figured that a bit more was going on here. We talked about this case in one of our seminars as an example of helping young adults who get into trouble as they try to leave home.

Despite Tim's resistance to taking credit for the positive outcomes he achieved with this case, our staff pressed on, urging Tim to tell the story about what he said and did with Butch and his parents that made things better. We asked Tim these mystery questions: How does a fortunate therapist like yourself seem to wind up in the right place at the right time so often with these difficult families, and keep getting these dramatic results? What can you tell us about your good fortune so that we might get lucky too? With this, Tim told us more about his conversations with Butch's family. Finally, we were able to put together some ideas about what went into the conversation with Butch and his parents that helped Butch to get sober and leave home. Over time, in close collaboration with Tim and another partner, Ken Russell, who also works extensively with mandated clients, we developed principles for how to work with these difficult cases.

When talking with mandated clients we must recognize that the social agencies involved have a problem that needs to be solved. Mandated clients can choose to meet or not meet with therapists. They can define a problem, or insist there is no problem and refuse to be involved in the evaluation or treatment. Still, the representative of the social agency has no other choice but to submit an evaluation to Family Court and make recommendations based on the client's compliance or resistance. Before speaking with the mandated client, it's helpful for therapists to contact the agency representatives and find out what their jobs impose on them. What are they required to do with the results of evaluation or treatment? How do they view the problem, the client, and the goals of therapy? What are their views of family members and influential others outside the family whose perceptions and actions shape the situation?

TALKING WITH A PROBATION OFFICER

Tim described his initial conversation with the probation officer (PO), Joan Tyler, as follows:

TYLER: Hi, Tim. I'd like to refer a 19-year-old young man for evaluation.

ADAMS: As part of his probation?

TYLER: I'm completing a PSI [presentence investigation] and his mother and I both think that alcohol is an issue for him.

ADAMS: What is he charged with?

TYLER: Assault. He threatened someone with a hammer and wound up in a fight with him. His mother has been worried about his drinking and thinks it's related. So do I. He seems basically like a good kid, but I think he might have a drinking problem.

ADAMS: Was he drinking at the time of this fight?

TYLER: No, he was driving and felt that another driver cut him off, so he and his friends pursued him to a stoplight, and he got out of the car with a hammer.

ADAMS: You're looking for an evaluation?

TYLER: Yes. If it's an issue, treatment will be part of my recommendation to the court. I think he'll need treatment, and I know you've had pretty good luck with kids like this.

ADAMS: He seems amenable?

TYLER: No, but he seems to have a close relationship with his mother. She and his stepfather seem very concerned, and I know you do a good job with families. So I thought of you. I hope it's more than an evaluation.

ADAMS: Are there any other complications, other people involved?

TYLER: No, not really. He has an attorney, but I think he'll agree with the mother that John needs his wings clipped.

ADAMS: It seems like everyone's on the same page, except John. Will he call me?

TYLER: I'll suggest that he do that.

ADAMS: I'll get back to you if he follows through. Thank you for thinking of me.

TYLER: Let me know if he makes an appointment.

ADAMS: Will do, ciao. [Tim always says "ciao" for some reason.]

ACKNOWLEDGING THE IMPOSITIONAL CONTEXT

Spurred on by his mother and probation officer, Butch called to arrange an appointment. In the first session, Butch came in reeking of cigarettes and stale beer, with bloodshot eyes and hair in wild disarray, looking like he had gotten about 2 hours sleep after partying all night. Butch expressed that it wasn't his idea to seek therapy. He was only there because he had to be. Typically, we suggest that the therapist state at the outset what he already knows about how the mandated client landed in therapy. Sharing this information allows the therapist to respect the impositional nature of the referral and highlight the key events linked to the requirement of treatment or evaluation.

If you know that parents had their children removed from the home, it's important to say you know. You can empathize with the parents' plight without taking sides about whether the children's removal was a good idea. If you know that someone lost their driver's license, acknowledge it and respect their experience of loss of freedom. In this case, Tim described what he knew about Butch's predicament, based on his conversation with the probation officer. Butch then filled in the details about how he became enraged when another driver pulled in front of him. He spoke about how the two drivers traded hand signals of an obscene nature, and admitted that he jumped out of the car with a hammer when he caught up with this driver at a stoplight. The two men fought until a bystander called the police, who arrested Butch for assault.

The therapist's next step was to inquire about whether Butch had been in therapy before. It's important to know the history of the mandated client's contact with helpers and helping agencies. Were there other occasions in which therapy was suggested or imposed? If so, by whom? If Butch was advised to seek professional help, what did Butch think about this advice?

ADAMS: Have you ever talked to a therapist?

BUTCH: No.

ADAMS: Has anyone ever suggested it before?

BUTCH: My mother.

ADAMS: Why?

BUTCH: She thinks I've got problems.

ADAMS: Like what?

BUTCH: She always has something to worry about, mostly drinking. She gets on me about things.

ADAMS: What kinds of things?

BUTCH: Just ... whatever ... she gets on me about things ... mostly drinking.

ADAMS: Is it okay with you that your mother gets on you?

BUTCH: No, the last thing I need is my mother worrying about me.

ADAMS: You don't want her to worry?

BUTCH: I don't want her watching everything I do, and I don't enjoy watching her worry.

ADAMS: It's not pretty?

BUTCH: My mother is basically a very nice person.

ADAMS: She means well.

BUTCH: Yes ...

ADAMS: So you never actually got to a therapist.

BUTCH: No, I never wanted to and, no offense, but I really don't want to talk with you.

Note how inquiries into the concern of others and the history of help seeking yields useful information about the problem. The conversation quickly shifts from Butch's views about therapy to the subject of drinking. We learn that Butch's mother has been worried about his drinking for some time and suggested therapy before. We find out that Butch doesn't like his mother watching over him. Nor would we guess he wants a probation officer looking into his business. We now have the makings of a mystery question. Why would a young man who doesn't like being scrutinized, behave in a way that leads to people watching and worrying?

ADAMS: I think we're in for it . . . not only have you never talked with someone about personal stuff, but now you're being forced to.

BUTCH: Yeah, it's kind of awkward.

ADAMS: And we've got to figure out how to talk to your probation officer . . . you and I need to get on track . . . to know how we're going to deal with these people around you.

BUTCH: What do you mean?

ADAMS: Well, it sounds like you've got all of these people, your PO, your mom, concerned about your drinking . . . it puts you and me in a funny position. You know your probation officer will ask you to sign a release.

BUTCH: She already did. I didn't sign it yet.

ADAMS: We've got an issue to deal with . . . most people come in here and put their best foot forward. Frankly, I congratulate you for coming in here really a mess, because you and I can be honest. You're obviously not trying to fool me . . . but we still have to figure out what to do with probation officers and mothers.

BUTCH: I thought you had to talk to her.

ADAMS: I can only release information with your permission.

BUTCH: So I don't have to sign the release?

ADAMS: No. You've been ordered to get an evaluation. You can do that with any qualified person your probation officer agrees to. It's important that you're comfortable talking with me and with what I tell your probation officer.

BUTCH: Can I decide what you tell her?

ADAMS: To an extent. I can report what I think about your drinking and how it affects you, or I can simply report some facts. Like you came here a certain number of times, for example.

BUTCH: You seem okay to talk to. What do we have to talk about?

Let's look briefly at the steps that Tim took to get to this point in the conversation. There were a number of possible approaches Tim could have taken when Butch arrived at his office unkempt and reeking of cigarettes and stale beer from the night before. Tim could have confronted Butch about how his appearance suggested he had a problem with alcohol. Tim could have enforced rules for proper interview behavior—ending the session and suggesting to Butch that he arrive alert for the next one. Or, Tim might have ignored Butch's appearance altogether. Instead, Tim made it clear that he noticed Butch's appearance, and that he was *not* going to watch over him. An important step in mandatory evaluation or treatment is for the therapist to distinguish his position from that of parent or probation officer.

Tim positioned himself as a conduit between Butch and the adults watching over him. He emphasized that Butch, too, was taking a clear position by being honest and not putting his best foot forward. Butch was not doing the standard things people do when they arrive for an evaluation interview—looking good, pulling the wool over the evaluator's eyes.

Tim suggested that despite social agency mandates, Butch still had personal agency. Butch had an opportunity to represent himself to the adults in his life in a variety of ways. The mandatory evaluation became a collaborative endeavor in which Butch and Tim together "figure[d] out what to do with probation officers and mothers." The conversation about confidentiality further clarified that Tim was not an agent of social control. Butch could decide whether information would be shared with his probation officer. Butch could even choose not to see Tim and select a different evaluator. Should Butch choose to meet with Tim, and give permission for Tim to send a report to the probation officer, Tim could report "just the facts," that Butch came to X sessions and they discussed Y, or he could present a thorough evaluation with clear recommendations. Tim suggested that he was interested in Butch's preferences for how he'd like to present himself to a probation officer who must do her job.

When Butch volunteered, "You seem okay to talk to," and asked, "What do we have to talk about?" he implied that he'd like an honest, in-depth evaluation. The conversation could then proceed much as it would for a voluntary client. Butch had invited Tim to assess the possibility of a drinking problem. They could figure out together how closely Butch wanted or needed to be monitored by adults in the context of this assessment.

A COLLABORATIVE INQUIRY ABOUT ALCOHOL USE

Tim started with the probation officer's views about a possible alcohol problem, respecting her position as definer of the problem and initiator of the evaluation. The inquiry into Butch's alcohol use proceeded.

ADAMS: Ms. Tyler thinks alcohol is a problem for you. What do you think she thinks about your drinking?

BUTCH: I think she wants me to prove to her that I won't drink again. She thinks I am f-ing up my life . . . that I'm a drunk. I wasn't even drinking when I had the fight.

ADAMS: Then why are people talking about alcohol?

BUTCH: Well, there were incidents.

ADAMS: Incidents?

BUTCH: I got tickets for drinking in public.

ADAMS: For drinking or being intoxicated?

BUTCH: Both.

ADAMS: And your PO . . . you're what, 19? . . . expects you to not drink for the rest of your life? That's pretty incredible. That would be a hard thing to do, wouldn't it?

BUTCH: Yeah, and I have no intention of stopping for the rest of my life.

ADAMS: It sounds like it's been a big part of your life. You were even out last night.

BUTCH: Yeah, I was.

ADAMS: Hey, alcohol and drugs are something that people do. It's a big part of people's lives. You seem to like it.

BUTCH: I do become the life of the party . . . I love a good time.

ADAMS: People would say you do it well?

Butch described how he *never* gets slobbering drunk or "stupid" or passes out. He described with pride how he maintains control while drinking "everyone under the table."

ADAMS: Some people get out of control . . . you don't?

BUTCH: No, I don't.

ADAMS: If I had three or four of your best friends here talking about your drinking, what would they say?

BUTCH: I can really pound them down.

ADAMS: No effect . . . alcohol usually affects people in some way.

BUTCH: Well, sometimes I get in fights.

ADAMS: Is that okay?

BUTCH: Yeah, I'd rather not be on probation though.

ADAMS: Think about this . . . I'd like to know how you'd like me to get back to your probation officer. You'd like people off your back. I'd like to work on that. I need something believable . . . saying that things are fine would only make people think you pulled the wool over my eyes. They'd probably send you to someone else. We could have a limited release . . . if there are some things you don't want to get back to your PO, it would allow me to say you were cooperative, uncooperative, working on issues . . . I can do that.

BUTCH: What's the other?

ADAMS: I'm not constrained. I can tell everything. You might want to think about what would work for you. The limited one might mean to her that you've got something to hide. If you're open and you're drinking, then she will know that. Think about it. We can talk more next time.

Butch arrived at the next session looking recently bathed and awake. In this less disoriented condition, Tim described Butch as a strikingly handsome kid—tall, dark-haired, with piercing green eyes and an affable demeanor. It was obvious to Tim that Butch would experience success on the party circuit and have no trouble attracting young women and a circle of cool friends. Being a "power drinker" was Butch's claim to fame during his teenage years. He was notorious where the local rowdies hung out, and this rowdy reputation followed him into his first year at college, where all he did was drink and party. But he knew that he was failing most of his subjects and "wasting his parents' hard earned money," so he dropped out and came back home.

In the second session, Tim asked a lot of preference questions about a range of topics including views of friends, family members, college, success, partying, popularity, being in therapy, and, of course, drinking alcohol. For example, Tim asked Butch how he felt about the incident with the hammer. Did he feel good about how he acted? Did he generally like it when he had an intimidating effect on people (like the other driver)? Did this give him a feeling of power? Did he think this incident enhanced his reputation with his friends? What was his mother's reaction to this incident and others like it? How did she regard him at this stage in his life? What did Butch think about his stepdad and stepbrother? What were their views about his situation? Was it a good thing that he was on probation? Did it feel comforting to have someone to check in with?

These questions were interspersed throughout a nonconfrontational, relaxed conversation that gave no appearance of a formal evaluation. Butch's responses to these questions helped Tim assemble a picture of preferred views. It became clear that Butch enjoyed being admired as someone who could control his drinking while still being the life of the party. But he didn't like being compared to some of his "drinking buddies." He said that many of them were "drunks," going nowhere, while his intention was to go to college and make something of himself. When Tim explored this preference for college, Butch said he was mad at himself for dropping out. He admitted that alcohol might not be helping him reach his goals. "Maybe I have a little bit of a problem with alcohol," he said. Butch talked more about his frustration at not having a clear plan for the future. He wanted to please his mother, but hadn't. He spoke with emotion about how he was often compared to his biological father, who bore his name. John Sr. was viewed by everyone in the family, including Butch, as a troubled alcoholic who spent time in jail on a variety of charges and abandoned his wife and son when Butch was quite young. Butch didn't like being seen as the spitting image of his father.

THE MYSTERY QUESTION WITH MANDATED CLIENTS

The mystery question for mandated clients assumes a typical form: How did a person with X preferred attributes (competent, independent, in control) wind up in Y position (being investigated by probation or Family Court, being scrutinized closely by other adults, being pressured to come for therapy)? Often, there's a wide gap between how mandated clients prefer to be seen (independent, autonomous) and how they describe their current predicament (watched closely by adults, having no freedom). Inviting clients to explain how they arrived in this troublesome fix is a resistance-proof way to obtain information about the evolution of the problem.

Vantage points	Butch
Preferred view of self	Attractive, popular, in control, responsible, different from my father.
View of significant others	My friends think I'm attractive. They see me as a partyer and power drinker.
View of family of origin	My mother is kind, generous. So is my stepfather. My father is irresponsible, reckless, alcoholic. **D.V.**—My parents think I'm bad, like my father.
View of therapist or other helpers	My probation officer (PO) thinks I need alcohol counseling. The evaluator (Tim) is interested in my opinions. He seems different from my PO.

FIGURE 15.1. Matrix of views.

Much of the conversation between Tim and Butch pivoted around the question of how an independent guy like Butch wound up in such a tight spot . . . being arrested, being investigated by a probation officer, and forced to come for therapy. After two sessions, Tim had a clear idea of how Butch wished to be seen as a person, how he viewed important others in his life (including alcohol), and how he saw those people seeing him. This information is summarized in the matrix of views (Figure 15.1).

Now clear about Butch's preferences and perspectives, Tim was ready to meet with the family. A similar version of the mystery question could now be posed to Butch's mother Marge and his stepfather James. In keeping with his wish to be honest and straightforward, Butch said that he wanted to talk about his views with his parents present in the room. Respecting Butch's preference, Tim invited Marge and James to attend the next session.

TALKING WITH FAMILY MEMBERS

In this family session, Tim engaged Butch, Marge, and James in a conversation about their family tree, which he drew on a blackboard for all to see. Objective assessments of family membership obtained through genograms of family trees can be used to fill out information in the matrix of views (the matrix is an assessment of family members' social constructions). When volatile problems such as alcohol abuse may be pulling families apart, orienting family members around a common task may bring them together. With this visual diagram of family membership to focus on, Tim invited the participants to comment on how they regarded the others on the tree. The person who drew the strongest emotional reaction from everyone was someone who wasn't even present. It was John Sr., Butch's biological father.

Marge's story about Butch's biological father filled in some of the blanks about how the configuration of the family (and the problem) evolved over time. She said that John Sr. walked out on the family when Butch was only 6 years old. Butch's contact with his father became sporadic over the years. John Sr. often made promises to come see his son that he'd fail to keep, and he would phone Butch at unpredictable times. Marge noticed that after these phone calls, Butch's behavior changed. He'd be angry and hard to manage. As he got older, Butch expressed more curiosity about his father and talked about wanting to see him.

When Butch was 12 years old, Marge remarried. James was very different from her first husband. He brought along a son who was the same age as Butch, and the two boys became close friends. Interestingly, no one in the group that now lived with each other had anything particularly negative to say about anyone else. Butch was fond of his stepbrother, Michael, and Michael was fond of him. Butch admired his stepdad, James, because he was responsible, caring, and generous to his mother, who he felt deserved to have good things happen to her. Marge said nice things about James and Michael. Everyone seemed to rank pretty high in everyone else's estimation except for Butch's own rating of himself. Butch felt like he stuck out like a sore thumb in this group of good people. Although he still lived inside the family, he acted more like the man outside the family who ranked the highest on the badness scale—John Anderson, Sr.

Butch's predicament at age 19 reminded us of the story of young Matt, who at age 7 said to the therapist (Tom), "When are we going to talk about it?" "What?" asked the therapist. "You know," Matt said, "that I'm bad." (See Chapter 8.) If you recall, Matt developed this unsettling idea of himself as a bad kid because he did bad things and wasn't stopped by his parents for doing them. Instead, his parents talked to him about how his bad behavior upset them, and they fretted about his jealousy toward his younger brother. Slowly and innocently, Matt's parents began acquiring the belief that Matt had "badness in him," and Matt picked up on this idea. Both the bad behavior and the negative self-image dissolved once Matt's parents calmly put a stop to the misbehavior, while also reassuring Matt that they regarded him as a good kid. Once Matt saw his parents unite to help him be the "good kid" he wished to be, he started to act in line with this preference, and they started to revise their troublesome view of him.

THE EVOLVING PROBLEM

In talking with Butch alone and then meeting with family members and hearing their stories, the following picture of the evolving problem emerged. Butch entered his adolescent years, as most children do, with concerns about who he was becoming. He had attributes that reminded everyone, including himself, of his father. He was handsome and charming; girls were drawn to him. He became popular and developed a reputation as a consummate "partyer." He experimented with alcohol and other substances, and tested parental limits by coming home late, often drunk. He soon discovered, as was the case in his younger years, that there were few parental limits. When Butch and his mother lived together, *he* decided when he would go to sleep at night, when to do his homework, and when to help out around the house. Although he and his mother were close in a conversational sense, he never regarded her as someone who would stop him from doing bad things. Butch and Marge were confidants, companions; he felt he could talk with her openly about almost anything and that she would do the same with him. Butch's stepdad, James, was a nice man, and Butch looked up to him. James was nothing like Butch's real father. He was kind, considerate, responsible, and reliable. He found he could talk to his stepfather just as he could to his mother, but James was also not inclined to set limits. As the teenage party scene became more intense, and the alcohol flowed freely, there were still no curfews, no homework-completion expectations, and no other responsibilities to perform at home. In a sense, Butch was permitted to be a "free spirit" during his teenage years. Yet his spirit kept drifting freely toward the ways of his father and away from the ways of his immediate family. Although Butch may have preferred to become more like his stepfather, he was acting more like his real father, and no one was stopping him.

The problem evolved as Butch came to see his parents regarding him as *like his father*, as he began acting like his father, as he affiliated with friends who admired these qualities that his father exuded, and as Marge and James tolerated these bad behaviors in him. The problem was maintained by too much talk and too little action, as Butch's parents did little to contain or limit his out-of-control behavior. The matrix of views (Figure 15.1), which reveals this narrative theme, became a guide to a helpful conversation.

In the next family session, Tim began by asking Marge to offer her explanation for Butch's current predicament. She said: "Butch has anger in him, and I think it runs pretty deep. I think it comes from his father walking out on the two of us, and his rejection of Butch over the years. I really think if he deals with the anger problem with you in therapy, the alcohol problem will take care of itself."

Butch responded by agreeing that he did have anger, but that he didn't think it came from his father. He explained that he was angry with himself for how he had been acting. "I need to have a job and a plan, and I need to just do it!" he said, sounding like a Nike commercial.

Butch's parents took notice of this statement of positive intention, probably because Butch had never spoken before with such conviction about his future. Yet, the statement wasn't surprising to Tim because Butch had already said similar things in their private conversations. Butch was now giving voice to his preferences in the presence of his parents and actively influencing their view of him.

Later in the conversation, Marge disclosed that she was worried that her son was becoming like his father. He was falling into the same behavior pattern that John Sr. showed in his adolescent years. With this, Butch bristled. "I'm *not* my father. I'm my own person." He then went on to say to his mother, "Sometimes I worry more about you being worried than anything else. I think it's time for me to start worrying for myself. I need to figure out who I am and what it is I want."

Tim then invited Butch's stepdad, James, to offer his opinion about the problem. James said that alcohol was the real problem, that Butch was addicted and he couldn't control himself. James felt that the anger came out because of the alcohol, disagreeing with Marge's view that the alcohol came out because of the anger. Butch listened respectfully, then presented his own view. "My father was—and is—an alcoholic," he said. "I'm not. I can stop anytime I want." (Having gleaned this information about family members' explanations and views, the matrix may be completed, as seen in see Figure 15.2.)

ARTICULATING PREFERENCES

In the context of this matrix of views, Tim was now in a maneuverable position to offer his own thoughts about what to do. He began by summarizing Butch's position about the problem. He recalled Butch's clearly stated preference to figure out what he wanted in life and accomplish it. He mentioned how Butch respected his mother and stepfather and was concerned about what they thought of him. Tim reviewed how Butch agreed with his mother that he was angry. He simply disagreed about the source of the anger. Butch said he was mad at himself for his own behavior, not because of his father. Tim noted how Butch also agreed with his stepfather about having a drink-

Vantage points	Butch	Marge	James
Preferred view of self	Attractive, popular, in control, responsible, different from my father.	Helpful, caring mother, compensating for irresponsible father.	Caring, competent stepfather, trying to be a good role model.
View of significant others	My friends think I'm attractive. They see me as a partyer and power drinker.	Butch is troubled, angry about being abandoned by his father. James is a good role model. Butch seems more like his biological father—reckless, angry. **D.V.**—Butch sees me as unhelpful.	Butch has an alcohol problem, like his biological father. Marge would like me to be helpful.
View of family of origin	My mother is kind, generous. So is my stepfather. My father is irresponsible, reckless, alcoholic. **D.V.**—My parents think I'm bad, like my father.		
View of therapist or other helpers	My probation officer (PO) thinks I need alcohol counseling. The evaluator (Tim) is interested in my opinions. He seems different from my PO.	Tim seems interested in my opinions. Perhaps he can help Butch with his anger.	Tim seems interested in my views. Perhaps he can help Butch with his drinking.

FIGURE 15.2. Complete matrix of views.

ing problem. Butch's view, however, was that he had control over his drinking. He could stop if he wanted to.

Tim then stated:

"While some alcohol counselors would strongly suggest that you attend AA at this time, I respect your position. I believe your intentions, and I see you as a very capable and determined person. You said clearly to me that you can stop drinking any time you put your mind to it. This seems like a good time to demonstrate that you're right, and to not touch alcohol in the 10 days between now and when we meet again. This way we can talk about the outcome, and we'll have some ideas about what the next step should be. This is not a success versus failure experiment. If you find out that you can't stop drinking, that'll give us some important information and we'll just take it from there."

Tim reiterated and supported Butch's stated preferences and intentions, and posed an experiment to answer the ongoing mystery question. The puzzling question now was as follows: Why would a young man who is capable and determined, clear about his preference to be different from his father (an alcoholic), angry at himself about his behavior, in control of whether or not he drinks alcohol, and interested in proving this to his parents, drink in the next 10 days? The results of this experiment to test self-control would determine how the conversation proceeded.

AN EXPERIMENT WITH SOBRIETY

Butch agreed to the challenge, and the family arrived 10 days later with news of sobriety.[1] Butch said he hadn't had a drink in 10 days and seemed proud of himself for sticking to his conviction. He refrained from going to parties during this time, because he felt he wasn't ready to deal with the pressure from friends. This experiment with sobriety led to more open conversations with the family about the past, present, and future. In subsequent discussions, Butch talked with his parents about the effects that alcohol had on his life and said with emotion that he was grateful to be alive. He referred to himself as a binge drinker and said that some of his binges could have cost him his life. He reminisced, for example, about two close friends who had been killed in an alcohol-related car crash that followed a party he was supposed to attend. He said that he could have been in that crash. There was also somber discussion between family members about John Sr.'s drinking and the devastating effects his behavior had on Butch and Marge. Butch began taking an antialcohol position as he conversed more and more about his life from a position of sobriety.

---

[1]It should be noted that Butch might have failed to demonstrate control of his drinking. In this instance, Butch's behavior would be out of sync with his stated preferences. This discrepancy could be explored in future conversation, not by characterizing the results as a failure, but by exploring the discrepancy with curiosity and interest. Perhaps, Butch would come to think of himself as out of control with his drinking, and so be more inclined to attend AA as a solution. By managing the conversation in a way that respects Butch's preferences, and holds him accountable to these preferences, different possibilities for solutions emerge.

Butch's experiment with sobriety continued as he committed himself to resisting the influence of alcohol in the weeks ahead. During this time, he came up with more severe tests of self-control by attempting to go to parties in which friends were drinking. He proved he could refuse alcohol and come home at a reasonable hour. As Butch's commitment to sobriety and his parents' confidence in his self-control increased, conversations about the "more important stuff" opened. On the subject of anger, Butch acknowledged that his mother was right, in part, about his resentment toward his father. He did feel rebuffed by him over and over again, and he was furious at him for the way he treated his mother. But he was also reviewing history in the context of his own present experiment with sobriety, and was now reframing his father's problem as an addiction problem, rather than a personal abandonment or rejection issue. Butch hoped that as he felt more in control of his own alcohol use, he could have a helpful conversation with his father about his father's alcohol use. Butch made it clear that he hadn't yet given up on having a relationship with his father.

COAUTHORING MANDATED REPORTS

Butch helped Tim figure out what to say in his report to the probation officer. Tim reported on Butch's recent sobriety, his attendance at weekly sessions, and his commitment to remain sober. As a result, the probation officer recommended a continuation of mandated counseling for 6 months and Butch's case was "ACD'd" (adjudicated in contemplation of dismissal), which meant that if he stayed sober and out of trouble for 6 months, the charges would be dropped.

On the subject of the future, Butch started looking into applying to colleges again and located a summer job away from home. He stuck to his "Nike proclamation," made in the family session, that it was time to "have a job, and a plan, and just do it." One family session was held during the summer to review progress. It appeared that Butch maintained sobriety, held on to his job, and saved money to put toward college. His plan to go back to college was in the works, and he was awaiting word from the three schools he'd applied to.

Butch was accepted at a small college in South Carolina for the winter quarter. He decided to move down to the area in the fall to look for a job. Since he had cousins living in the community, he figured they would help him find a place to live and locate employment. Also, Butch's father lived only 2 hours away from the campus and Butch planned to contact him. This plan for reaffiliation with his father set off alarms in Marge and James who expressed concern that being in close proximity to John Sr. would make it more difficult for Butch to continue in his independent, responsible, and sober ways. Butch said that he hoped to present himself to his father as someone who had changed and was doing positive things with his life. This clear statement of positive intention reassured the parents somewhat, but they remained skeptical.

FUTURE TALK

Tim's position about the future was that "the jury was still out on the subject of drinking." The temptation to binge and party on campus would be great, and it remained to be seen how much control Butch would have over himself. Tim left Butch with a host of questions to ponder that would help him monitor his own progress. Although these questions were not posed in the exact manner or sequence described, the following kinds of issues were raised by Tim in conversation with Butch: How will you know when you get into trouble with alcohol again, Tim asked? What would be the telltale signs? How will it be for you to encounter your father with sober eyes and notice the difference between you? When you see your dad, will you feel disloyal about having become more like your mom and stepdad? How will it be to part company with the person you were named after, and look so much like? How will you evaluate your parents' concerns about the negative effects of living near your father? With proximity, will you feel more under your father's influence, your parents', or your own? It may take strong commitment to show your father that you're your own man. It may take resilience to weather another rebuff from him if he sees that you're doing better than he is.

These are future-oriented *inoculation questions* and comments. They prepare Butch to consider different likely possibilities and appeal to him to keep monitoring and evaluating his own position about future events. Also, probable events such as rejection by his father are reframed in the context of difference between them. Butch is encouraged to continue to consider whether he prefers to live life like his father, or not, as he moves into adulthood.

As seems to be the custom with a number of the young people Tim has talked with over the years, they keep in touch. Butch called halfway into his first semester to say that things were still going well. When Tim got in touch with Marge and James at a later date, they said they remained pleased with Butch's progress and passed on a recent message from Butch. "Say hi to Tim," they said. (It seemed somehow that we had heard that phrase before.)

WHEN THERAPY ISN'T ENOUGH

In many instances, therapy with mandated clients doesn't go as smoothly as it did with Butch and his family. Often, clients indicate directly or indirectly that they're not in control of their drinking, their tempers, or their children. They may continue to arrive late for sessions or simply not show up. They may not say with conviction, as Butch did, that they prefer to be responsible and in charge of their own lives. In these instances, the therapist/evaluator would provide this information to the person monitoring the client's behavior and suggest that the client was not likely to take responsibility for his or her own behavior through therapy alone.

The principles of helpful conversation apply, however, even in these less than ideal circumstances. It's the therapist's job to investigate *how social control evolved* in the lives of mandated clients and their families. It's not the therapist's job to assume a position of social control or to advocate against the intrusion of social agencies. If the therapist maintains a respectful position and invites the client's preferences and views about self and others, even recommendations for social control can accommodate preferred views. Believe it or not, we've engaged in many conversations with mandated clients in which biological parents ultimately acknowledge that their children are better off remaining with foster parents until the intense conflict that now rules family life subsides. As the biological parents cooperate with the foster parents and children perceive unity in the adult world, future solutions become possible.

We've also spoken with men mandated for treatment following incidents of family violence who decide that they themselves benefit from the social control of an Order of Protection now filed with Family Court. These men acknowledge that the Court Order, which now prevents them from speaking with partners and children, is a good idea. This acknowledgment emerges after the therapist asks a series of preference questions, much as Tim did with Butch. The mandated client says, in essence, that he'd like to be in control of his own emotions so that he might someday be perceived by his wife and children as capable and responsible. The therapist then asks the man to predict what he thinks would happen if he were free to talk with his wife and a controversial topic were to come up. The man says that he could easily explode, that there's no telling what he might do. As the conversation progresses, the man decides that the Order of Protection actually protects *him* from acting in a way that violates his own preferences. Thus, the therapist sends a report to Family Court recommending that the Order of Protection be continued, along with therapy. Since the report reflects the preferences of the mandated client, there's little resistance to the therapist's recommendations. In this way, even reports that advocate social control can be coauthored, increasing the likelihood of compliance with court orders. What was once impositional becomes voluntary.

The principal goal in working with mandated clients is to encourage their personal agency in figuring out how and in what ways social agencies fit into the fabric of their lives. If social controls do fit with the client's preferred narrative account, then these controls may need to stay in place. However, if mandated clients, such as Butch, decide to regain personal control of their lives and relationships, practical solutions can be reached. Helping mandated clients take action to live their lives responsibly, without the costly supervision of social control agencies, is a particularly rewarding aspect of our work.

—16—

Back to the Future

In the Introduction, we posed the following questions that oriented our conversation with you, the reader: What are the key ingredients of a helpful conversation? What gets said in the therapy room that so alters the patterns of meaning and action in people's lives? What inspires people to talk with each other differently and steers them toward solutions?

We asked these questions as we reflected on what worked in a conversation between Tom and an overwhelmed stepfather named Vern. Vern was caught up in a problematic way of looking at his 13-year-old stepson's recent misbehavior. He saw Timmy as disrespecting his authority, which led him to apply military school tactics. Vern felt that his wife, Alice, disapproved of his harsh approach, and along with Timmy, regarded him in a negative light. Vern persisted in these tactics despite the fact that the approach wasn't working. From Vern's point of view, Alice and Timmy had teamed up against him. As Tom spoke with Vern, and Alice and Joe looked on, Vern transformed before their eyes into a different-looking and different-talking person.

In the room, Vern changed from being a man who sat back in his chair and defended his harsh discipline tactics with tight-lipped rage into a man who sat forward in his chair and proclaimed with warm enthusiasm his new commitment to be "nice to the boy." At home, Vern set about to revive the loving relationship he'd once had, and always wanted to have, with Timmy. Alice, who withdrew from Vern during the drill sergeant era, welcomed this new stage in family life. Vern and Alice became partners again.

You may recall another vignette from one of our case stories—that of Al, who became depressed in his later years after developing emphysema (Chapter 13). Al, too, transformed in the therapy room. In the first session, Al was a person who spoke hesitantly and sadly about his failed effort to shovel snow under the influence of emphysema. By the fifth session, he spoke confidently about a new conversation he'd had with his family about the facts of his illness and how he intended to manage it. Similar shifts in the ambience of conversation, inside and outside the therapy room, have been described throughout this book. Let's review our response to this question of what makes a therapeutic conversation therapeutic.

The art of developing narrative solutions is a little like the art of writing. Like good writers, skilled narrative therapists rearrange life images and scenes that link the past, present, and future. In describing the life work of Virginia Woolf, literary commentator Ruth Miller (1981) observed how Woolf frequently used the images of rooms, mirrors, windows, and thresholds to portray how her characters framed their experience. Woolf drew the reader into a character's current frame of reference—within the enclosed space of the room or the eclipsed view outside the window—then, subtly, shifted away from this frame to other images.

Consider this image from the story "A Lady in the Looking Glass," in which Woolf draws the reader into the experience of looking at letters that have fallen onto a table underneath a mirror:

> There they lay on the marble topped table, all dripping with light and colour at first and crude and unabsorbed. And then it was strange to see how they were drawn in and arranged and composed and made part of the picture and granted that stillness and immortality which the looking-glass conferred. They lay there invested with a new reality and significance and with greater heaviness, too, as if it would have needed a chisel to dislodge them from the table. And, whether it was fancy or not, they seemed to have become not merely a handful of casual letters but to be tablets graven with eternal truth—if one could read them, one would know everything to be known about Isabella, yes, and about life, too. (quoted in Miller, 1981, p. 2)

The illusion created was one of "knowing Isabella" through these letters etched within the looking glass. The narrative device of the looking glass, however, reminded the reader that he or she was reflecting only upon a slice of Isabella's life through the mirror on the table. As the writer shifted to other stories and images of Isabella, the reader learned that the reflection through the glass did not represent a complete picture of Isabella's life. To know her, we needed to be acquainted with other scenes and images.

The room was another metaphor used by Virginia Woolf to depict the concept of frame. In the confines of their rooms, Woolf's characters were protected from the unpredictable events that occurred in the world outdoors. The room created a boundary that somehow held these uncontrollable forces at bay. Consider this passage from the novel *Jacob's Room*, in which a family was depicted sitting at a dinner table, safe from the world outside the room:

> Here, inside the room, seemed to be order and dry land; there, outside, a reflection in which things wavered and vanished, waterily . . . and they were all conscious of making a party together in a hollow, on an island; had their common cause against that fluidity out there. (quoted in Miller, 1981, p. 78)

In the narrative solutions approach, the therapist unravels the mystery of how people construct the closed-in frames that constrict their experience in order to know how to guide the conversation into the "fluidity out there." Let's return to a scene from Al's story.

SCENES FROM A ROOM

In the first session, Al told a story that depicted a scene from his current life. It was a late January afternoon, and he was gazing out the window from what had become his familiar despondent perch, the living room couch. There he caught a glimpse of his agile 25-year-old son swiftly removing the snow from the driveway that he (Al) labored so hard to shovel away that morning. This image from the room was only a snapshot from Al's life, yet it came to represent who he felt he now was, and who he believed he was becoming.

The therapist created movement away from the closed-in frame of the living room by shifting Al's focus to other snapshots from his life. Al recalled occasions when he was able to set realistic limits, to stay connected with family, to remain active and useful even when constrained and challenged. It was then that he was able to reorient himself to the present and develop a different picture of the future.

THRESHOLDS

In Woolf's writing, the threshold symbolized that encapsulated moment in time when people pause before moving through an important transition in life. As Miller (1981) noted, "a scene at a threshold lends itself to symbolic interpretations not only because it is framed but also because it occurs at a point at which time is suspended" (p. 89). A passage from Woolf's novel *To the Lighthouse* depicted a main character, Mrs. Ramsay, pausing on her way out of the dining room:

It was necessary now to carry everything a step further. With her foot on the threshold she waited a moment longer in a scene which was vanishing even as she looked, and then, as she moved and took Minta's arm and left the room, it changed, it shaped itself differently; it had become, she knew, giving one last look at it over her shoulder, already the past. (quoted in Miller, 1981, pp. 172–173)

With that "step further," Mrs. Ramsay left the past and entered the future. According to Miller (1981), the pause at the threshold was a way to extend the present to make life stand still (p. 89). As people cross through important thresholds in life, they sometimes stumble, then step into problems. They lose their forward momentum.

As Rachel crossed the threshold from childhood into adolescence (Chapters 6 and 7), she was labeled "incorrigible." The scenes in Rachel's life that were now noticed involved fights in the schoolyard. Transfixed by these scenes, Rachel's teachers, principal, classmates, and, finally, her mother, lost sight of who Rachel was and wanted to become. Her life was framed negatively by people important to her, and her rebellious behavior kept supporting that frame.

When Carl (Chapter 11) left his parents' home, crossing the threshold into adulthood, he lost confidence in his abilities. After three experiences of failure in different colleges, Carl recrossed the threshold back into his parents' home and was received as a different person. The current scenes from Carl's life were now confined to the interior of that home from which he rarely ventured forth. Soon, Carl and his parents focused in on a frame of failure in which only Carl's laziness was noticed, and his ambition obscured from view.

Valerie set forth from her parents' home, went off to college and performed well there (Chapter 11). It wasn't until she fell in love for the first time, and experienced conflict in this new relationship, that she relived scenes from her past. Valerie developed symptoms that she'd once had when she was only 9 years old and witnessed conflict in her parents' marriage. Not knowing how to manage conflict in her new relationship, these old symptoms returned. Now Valerie began noticing the cracks in the sidewalks, which slowed her movement to and from her classes. She fixed her attention on the words on the pages of her school books as she read them over and again, trying futilely to complete her homework. Soon, time stood still. Valerie's plans to complete college were now in doubt, her confidence in her new relationship was shaken, and her forward movement in life suspended.

When Al crossed the threshold into his later years, it wasn't his chronological age or the recent retirement from his job that stopped him in his tracks. It was the event of major illness that altered the forward trajectory of his life. Emphysema brought with it not only the confinement of physical limitations but also the constraints of self-doubt. Al started to question who he now was and who he was becoming.

THE PAIN OF DISJUNCTION

As people cross thresholds in life, they're apt to look around and see how they appear through the eyes of others. As Al peered through the window at his youthful son shoveling snow outdoors, a life spectrum of images may have crossed his mind. There was the present image of his son completing the snow shoveling job that Al had failed to finish earlier that day. There was the past image of himself as a son watching his father grow idle and unproductive as he withered under the influence of illness. There was the present image of Al's son reflecting on him lying there motionless on the couch—thinking of Al as Al had once thought of his own father. There was the future image of himself becoming more and more useless to family members who rarely consulted him about their needs and concerns.

Perhaps it was the intersection of all these images that resulted in the pained look that the therapist saw on Al's face as he told the snow-shoveling story. A century ago, William James, a psychologist living within a family of writers, captured the experience of the pain of disjunction in a memorable way:

> Those images of me in the minds of other men are, it is true, things outside of me, whose changes I perceive just as I perceive any other outward change. But the pride and shame which I feel are not concerned merely with *those* changes. I feel as if something else had changed too, when I perceive my image in your mind to have changed for the worse, something in me to which that image belongs, and which a moment ago I felt inside of me, big and strong and lusty, but now weak, contracted, and collapsed. (1890/1984, p. 97)

ONCE UPON A TIME BEFORE THE PROBLEM BEGAN

We bring to conversations with people in distress a curiosity about how the present problem became a problem. This curiosity pervades the therapeutic conversation from beginning to end. It's a curiosity that becomes contagious, that spreads to the people touched by the problem, who are grappling for solutions. Clients become curious themselves about how they came to construct this seemingly fixed reality called the problem. They puzzle with us over how they came to act in ways they don't like and to see each other in ways that violate their preferences.

The therapeutic conversation creates images that "waver and vanish, waterily," as in Virginia Woolf's passage about the room. The image of Carl as a lazy young man who refuses to step outside the family home now mingles with images of Carl as ambitious, as burning to succeed like his parents. Soon family members converse about how to help Carl recapture this ambition gone awry so that he gets moving again.

The scene that Al witnessed outside the living room window takes new form (and meaning) when he recalls his past successes in managing adversity and setting realistic limits. Perhaps he wasn't observing a son taking over for a useless old man. Perhaps there is still "fluidity out there" in the world outdoors and a chance to participate in that world.

Fairy tales often begin with the line, "Once upon a time. . . ." As we inquire into the preproblem past with interest, clients may recount alternative stories that cast new light on their present experience. These once-upon-a-time stories, however, aren't fairy tales made up by therapists to help people feel better about their lives. They are actual accounts of life experience imparted by clients. As therapists listen intently to these accounts, they may see that events not too different from those now occurring, were once managed differently by people involved in the problem. The stories that get told in response to our inquiries about life without the problem often reveal strengths inherent in people to resolve the problem. Narrative solutions emerge when people envision the past, present, and future of their lives in ways that confirm their strengths and preferences.

Virginia Woolf notwithstanding, while there are *poetical* features to this narrative solutions approach that continue to intrigue us, today's cost-conscious times demand *practical* solutions. The practice of psychotherapy in the United States has changed dramatically under the influence of managed care. Therapists of different schools and persuasions are being challenged to shorten the length of therapy, account for outcomes, and demonstrate that their approaches are cost-effective. Psychotherapists are more aware than ever that health-care dollars are not without limits, that efficiency matters.

The narrative solutions approach is based in the practical, parsimonious tradition of the MRI brief therapy approach. Over the course of this book, we've described practical solutions to a range of different problems that present at different stages in the life cycle. In almost all of the cases presented, therapy was brief, between 3 and 15 sessions.

Although the narrative solutions approach is generally brief, it also may be applied to problems that require longer term treatment. For example, the case of "Sam's Secret" (Chapter 12) demonstrated how our approach worked to resolve a tenacious problem that had enduring impact on a young man's self-concept.

Stories of sexual abuse that remain locked away and rarely, if ever, circulated in conversations with others, have holding power in shaping negative views of self. Since it takes time and trust for people to reveal experiences of trauma and subjugation, let alone to reconsider how they have shaped their lives and supported problems, therapy is often not short term.

Therapists need to take ample time to listen, understand, connect with preferred views, and help clients rethink their assumptions about self and others in the context of such silent yet powerful narratives. These are not cases in which therapists should feel pressured to resolve problems in 10 sessions or less.

You'll recall that due to the therapist's trusted other position, Sam returned to therapy at significant junctures in his adult life, well after his presenting symptoms improved. Sam talked with the therapist after he married, then during his wife's pregnancy, then again after the birth of the couple's first child. Sam initiated these conversations to consolidate narrative solutions—to ensure that he maintained the intimacy he now cherished with his wife, and to bolster his confidence about being the father he hoped to be. Sam's periodic reentries into therapy did not signify that he was becoming too dependent on the therapist. This intermittent-conversations approach became a way for Sam to expand upon the trust he developed with the therapist so that he could develop trust in new relationships. Gradually, in the wake of new conversations outside the therapy room, the story of sexual abuse lost its holding power on Sam's identity.

The narrative solutions approach provides a framework for cost-effective therapy based on a model of resilience rather than deficit. The emphasis is on *what's strong in people, not on what's wrong in people*. How long therapy takes depends on the availability of resources within and between people, and a therapist's ability to access these resources through helpful conversations. Therapy can often be brief, even when presenting symptoms are severe or persist over a long period of time.

The case of Valerie (Chapter 11), who presented with severe symptoms of OCD is a case in point. Soon into the therapeutic conversation, the therapist realized that a key resource available to Valerie was that she was free from these intrusive symptoms for most of her life. Valerie also showed competence and resilience in many areas—academic success, organizational know-how, sensitivity to others, and responsibility. Valerie's symptoms improved dramatically in only five sessions as she figured out how these negative thoughts and compulsions evolved and what she needed to do to keep her symptoms at bay.

In contrast to Valerie's OCD symptoms, Helen's hives were chronic and persistent throughout her adolescent and adult life (Chapter 13). Helen, too, had other stories to tell about her life experience that didn't fit with the story of hives. For example, she spoke about her resilience in leaving an unhappy marriage in which her own voice was submerged, her wisdom in forming a new relationship with a man who valued her ideas, and her enduring determination to conduct her life differently from that of her own mother (who also suffered hives). By exploring these preferred narrative accounts and examining the mystery of hives in the context of Helen's strengths, Helen figured out what to do to eliminate these troublesome symptoms. In Helen's case, lifelong hives improved over 10 sessions and resolved in a matter of 20 sessions conducted intermittently within a 1-year period.

Not only is the narrative solutions approach cost-effective in treating a range of clinical problems that present at different developmental stages, but the approach also applies to helpful conversations outside the therapy room. The same principles for how to conduct helpful conversations with family members also apply in talking effectively with caseworkers from departments of social services, probation officers, teachers, guidance counselors, attorneys, law guardians, judges, and other professionals whose views and actions impact on the lives of clients.

The extrapolation of narrative solution concepts to working with mandated clients, such as Butch (Chapter 15), and families embroiled in intense conflict, such as Sally's family (Chapter 14), has helped our practice grow in new and exciting directions. At CFI, we have treatment, evaluation, and consultation contracts with public and private agencies. Our aim is to help people who become involved with social agencies, including people who are told they have to talk with us.

THE EXCITEMENT OF AN INTEGRATIVE APPROACH

Another satisfying aspect of the narrative solutions approach is that it integrates ideas that transcend divisions between schools of psychotherapy. In this approach, therapists can meet with individuals, yet still think about changing interactional patterns. Therapists can alter meanings with the goal in mind of changing behavior. Therapists can be collaborative, respectful, and nonimpositional in their approach, while still being purposeful and planful. Therapists can talk about problems while still promoting solutions. Therapists can track how problems evolve to obtain clues to how problems resolve. Therapists can change present patterns and shift future perspectives by focusing on people's past experiences. Therapists can use the techniques of restorying and reframing together. Therapists can be brief and practical while embracing the poetical aspects of the human experience. Therapists can work effectively with voluntary clients who request their help, as well as with mandated clients who talk with them because they have to.

Along with these elements of integration come exciting opportunities for using skills not often linked to doing narrative or brief therapy. Therapists can be empathetic and nonjudgmental without thinking that they're being idle. Empathetic reflection isn't about sitting expressionless in a chair and saying, "Umm," or, "Ah-hah," to the important things clients say. When narrative solutions therapists empathize by connecting with preferred views, they're implementing a key component of an action plan. Solutions develop as clients see others (including therapists) seeing them in preferred ways.

Narrative solutions therapists can also incorporate knowledge about normal developmental processes into therapeutic conversations. Knowing where children are in their cognitive and emotional maturation informs how therapists talk with children. This knowledge also affects how therapists talk with parents about how to talk with children. Knowing about how adolescents' strivings for independence couple with their unspoken need for parental guidance helps in planning helpful conversations between defiant teenagers and their parents. Knowing that women in our culture are taught to think of the needs of others while submerging their own preferences helps in steering conversations with young women who experience life-threatening eating problems. This knowledge also helps in talking with parents about how to help their adolescent daughters nurture a self-orientation. Knowing that young adults can often develop symptoms at the point in time that they leave their parents' homes, or during the stage of forming intimate partnerships, helps guide our conversations with young adults. Knowing that older adults reminisce about their pasts, and compare historical accounts to present experiences, helps in figuring out how to empower older adults. We can bring the past back to life to change present thoughts and actions, and alter future perspectives.

Narrative solutions therapists can incorporate innovations and techniques from other schools of therapy without feeling that they're being disloyal to their own theoretical approach. For example, the technique of externalizing, developed by narrative therapist Michael White, fits with the theoretical underpinnings of this approach. Externalizing conversations encourage people to talk about problems in ways that separate themselves from the problem's effects. Thus, externalizing conversations may confirm preferred views of self and narrow disjunctive gaps that propel people into problems. Solution-focused techniques such as the miracle question also fit comfortably within a narrative solutions approach. As people describe a future vision of life without the problem, they give us clues about how they prefer to view themselves, and depict modes of behavior that fit within their own preferences. Therapists may ask miracle questions along with mystery questions in managing helpful conversations with families.

We've described several cases in this book in which skills and techniques developed outside the field of family therapy were incorporated in the service of narrative solutions. Of all things, dream analysis was used to help Sam reconstruct the meaning of recurrent nightmares. No doubt, Sigmund Freud would squirm at this social constructionist approach to dreams, yet Sam was helped to reconstruct the meaning of dreams in a way that confirmed his preferences and positive intentions. You may also recall that Valerie (Chapter 11) did her own version of dream analysis when she reframed recent nightmares as meaning that she was now more in touch with her own thoughts and emotions. Psychoeducational assessment techniques were used with a 10-year-old boy named Jeff (Chapter 8) to help understand the nature of his difficulties in school. This objective assessment not only led to the detection of a seizure disorder, but also helped Jeff's parents reconcile differences in perception about Jeff's capabilities. Equipped with new knowledge about Jeff, parents once in conflict pulled together to build his confidence.

Perhaps the most important aspect of integration in this work is that narrative solutions are linked to the broad spectrum of life experience that speaks to who we are and what we are capable of. At its core, this brief therapy approach is about bringing out the best in people.

References

Andersen, T. (1991). *The reflecting team: Dialogues & dialogues about the dialogues.* New York: Norton.

Anderson, H., & Goolishian, M. A. (1992). The client is the expert: A not knowing approach to therapy. In K. J. Gergen & S. McNamee (Eds.), *Therapy as a social construction* (pp. 25–39). Newbury Park, CA: Sage.

Bateson, G. (1972). *Steps to an ecology of mind.* New York: Ballantine.

Bateson, G. (1988). *Mind and nature.* New York: Bantam.

Berg, I. K., & de Shazer, S. (1993). Making numbers talk: Language in therapy. In S. Friedman (Ed.), *The new language of change* (pp. 5–24). New York: Guilford Press.

Bogdan, J. (1986). Do families really need problems? Why I am not a functionalist. *Family Therapy Networker, 10*(4), 30–35, 67–69.

Boscolo, L., Cecchin, G., Hoffman, L., & Penn, P. (1987). *Milan systemic therapy.* New York: Basic Books.

Carter, B., & McGoldrick, M. (Eds.). (1980). *The changing family life cycle: A framework for family therapy.* New York: Gardner Press.

Carter, B., & McGoldrick, M. (1989). Overview the changing family life cycle: A framework for family therapy. In B. Carter & M. McGoldrick (Eds.), *The changing family life cycle: A framework for family therapy* (2nd ed., pp. 3–28). Boston: Allyn & Bacon.

Combrinck-Graham, L. (1989). Family models of childhood psychopathology. In L. Combrinck-Graham (Ed.), *Children in family contexts* (pp. 67–89). New York: Guilford Press.

Coyne, J. C. (1985). Toward a theory of frames and reframing: The social nature of frames. *Journal of Marital and Family therapy, 11,* 337–344.

de Shazer, S. (1985). *Keys to solutions in brief therapy.* New York: Norton.

de Shazer, S. (1991). *Putting difference to work.* New York: Norton.

Efran, J. S., & Clarfield, L. E. (1992). Constructivist therapy: Sense and nonsense. In S. McNamee & K. J. Gergen (Eds.), *Therapy as social construction* (pp. 200–217). London: Sage.

Efran, J. S., Lukens, R. J., & Lukens, M. D. (1988). Constructivism: What's in it for you? *Family Therapy Networker, 12*(5), 27–35.

Eron, J., & Lund, T. W. (1989). From magic to method: Principles of effective reframing. *Family Therapy Networker, 13*(1), 64–68, 81–83.

Eron, J. B., & Lund, T. W. (1993). How problems evolve and dissolve: Integrating narrative and strategic concepts. *Family Process, 32*, 291–309.

Fisch, R., Weakland, J. H., & Segal, L. (1982). *The tactics of change: Doing therapy briefly*. San Francisco: Jossey-Bass.

Garcia-Preto, N. (1989). Transformation of the family system in adolescence. In B. Carter & M. McGoldrick (Eds.), *The changing family life cycle: A framework for family therapy* (2nd ed., pp. 255–283). Boston: Allyn & Bacon.

Gergen, K. (1985). The social constructionist movement in modern psychology. *American Psychologist*. 40:266–275.

Gilligan, C. (1982). *In a different voice: Psychological theory and women's development*. Cambridge, MA: Harvard University Press.

Goffman, E. (1974). *Frame analysis: An essay on the organization of experience*. Boston: Northeastern University Press.

Goolishian, H., & Anderson, H. (1987). Language systems and therapy: An evolving idea. *Psychotherapy, 24*, 529–538.

Haley, J. (1973). *Uncommon therapy*. New York: Norton.

Haley, J. (1976). *Problem solving therapy*. San Francisco: Jossey-Bass.

Haley, J. (1980). *Leaving home: The therapy of disturbed young people*. New York: McGraw-Hill.

Haley, J. (Ed.). (1985a). *Conversations with Milton H. Erickson, M.D.: Vol. 1. Changing individuals*. Rockville, MD: Triangle Press.

Haley, J. (Ed.). (1985b). *Conversations with Milton H. Erickson, M.D.: Vol. 2. Changing couples*. Rockville, MD: Triangle Press.

Haley, J. (Ed.). (1985c). *Conversations with Milton H. Erickson, M.D.: Vol 3. Changing children and families*. Rockville, MD: Triangle Press.

James, W. (1984). The principles of psychology. In B. W. Wiltshire (Ed.), *William James: The essential writings* (pp. 44–161). Albany: SUNY Press. (Original work published 1890)

Jones, C. W. (1986). Frame cultivation: Helping new meanings take root in families. *American Journal of Family Therapy, 14*, 57–68.

Laing, R. D. (1960). *The divided self*. London: Tavistock.

Laing, R. D. (1969). *Self and others*. London: Tavistock.

Laing, R. D. (1970). *Knots*. London: Tavistock.

Laing, R. D., Phillipson, H., & Lee, A. R. (1966). *Interpersonal perceptions: A theory and method of research*. London: Tavistock.

Madanes, C. (1980). The prevention of re-hospitalization of adolescents and young adults. *Family Process, 19*, 179–192.

Madanes, C. (1990). *Sex, love and violence: Strategies for transformation*. New York: Norton.

Maddi, S. (1968). *Personality theories: A comparative analysis*. Homewood, IL: Dorsey Press.

Markus, H., & Nurius, P. (1986). Possible selves. *American Psychologist, 41*, 954–969.

Miller, R. C. (1981). *Virginia Woolf: The frames of art and life*. New York: St. Martin's Press.

Minuchin, S. (1974). *Families and family therapy*. Cambridge, MA: Harvard University Press.

Minuchin S., & Fishman, H. C. (1981). *Family therapy techniques*. Cambridge, MA: Harvard University Press.

Minuchin, S., Rosman, B. L., & Baker, L. (1978). *Psychosomatic families: Anorexia nervosa in context*. Cambridge, MA: Harvard University Press.

Nichols, M. P. (1987). *The self in the system: Expanding the limits of psychotherapy*. New York: Brunner/Mazel.

Nichols, M. P. (1995). *The lost art of listening*. New York: Guilford Press.

Rogers, C. R. (1951). *Client centered therapy*. Boston: Houghton Mifflin.

Rogers, C. R. (1961). *On becoming a person: A therapist's view of psychotherapy*. Boston: Houghton Mifflin.

Rohrbaugh, M., & Eron, J. B. (1982). The strategic systems therapies. In L. E. Abt & R. I. Stuart (Eds.), *The newer therapies: A workbook* (pp. 248–266). New York: Van Nostrand Reinhold.

Selvini Palazzoli, M., Boscolo, L., Cecchin, G., & Prata, G. (1978). *Paradox and counterparadox*. New York: Jason Aronson.

Shirk, S. R. (1983). *Self evaluation and self doubt in adolescence: A social cognitive analysis*. Unpublished doctoral dissertation, New School for Social Research, New York.

Tomm, K. (1984a). One perspective on the Milan Systemic Appproach: Part I. Overview of development, theory and practice. *Journal of Marital and Family Therapy, 10*, 113–125.

Tomm, K. (1984b). One perspective on the Milan Systemic Approach: Part II. Description of session format, interviewing style and interventions. *Journal of Marital and Family Therapy, 10*, 253–271.

Watzlawick, P. (1976). *How real is real?* New York: Random House.

Watzlawick, P. (1978). *The language of change*. New York: Basic Books.

Watzlawick, P. (Ed.). (1984). *The invented reality*. New York: Norton.

Watzlawick, P., Beavin, J. H., & Jackson, D. D. (1967). *Pragmatics of human communication*. New York: Norton.

Watzlawick, P., & Coyne, J. C. (1980). Depression following stroke: Brief problem-focused family treatment. *Family Process, 19*, 13–18.

Watzlawick, P., Weakland, J., & Fisch, R. (1974). *Change: Principles of problem formation and problem resolution*. New York: Norton.

Weakland, J. (1995). Letter to the editor. *Family therapy Networker, 19*(5), 16.

Weakland, J. H., Fisch, R., Watzlawick, P., & Bodin, A. M. (1974). Brief therapy: Focused problem resolution. *Family Process, 13*, 141–168.

White, M. (1989). *Selected papers*. Adelaide, Australia: Dulwich Centre Publications.

White, M., & Epston, D. (1990). *Narrative means to therapeutic ends*. New York: Norton.

Index

DATE DUE			
APR 0 7 1997			
NOV 2 9 1999			